Universal praise for *The FastDiet*

"The biggest diet revolution since Atkins."

—Daily Mail (London)

"The only diet you'll ever need."

—Mail on Sunday (London)

"I have several patients who have started to successfully follow the diet and think it is wonderful."

—Dr. Pete Bridgwood

"Thank you, Michael, for bringing this leading-edge science to our attention. We now feel in control of our health and weight for the first time in many years, and I'm committed to continuing the program for life. I hope everyone gets to know about this. You deserve a knighthood!"

—Brian M., dieter

"My partner and I have been on the diet and have each lost about 10 pounds without too much hardship."

—Claire Cronin, dieter

"I've followed the diet ever since watching Michael Mosley's TV program. It's radically changed my attitude to food/hunger, I feel more energetic, and losing nearly 15 pounds has been a delightful plus. It was the science that interested me. I know an amazing amount of other people who also wouldn't 'diet' but who are intermittent fasting. I actually value the fasting days in a way I never thought I would, which makes them easy to stick to. I don't intend to ever drop it."

—Susie White, dieter

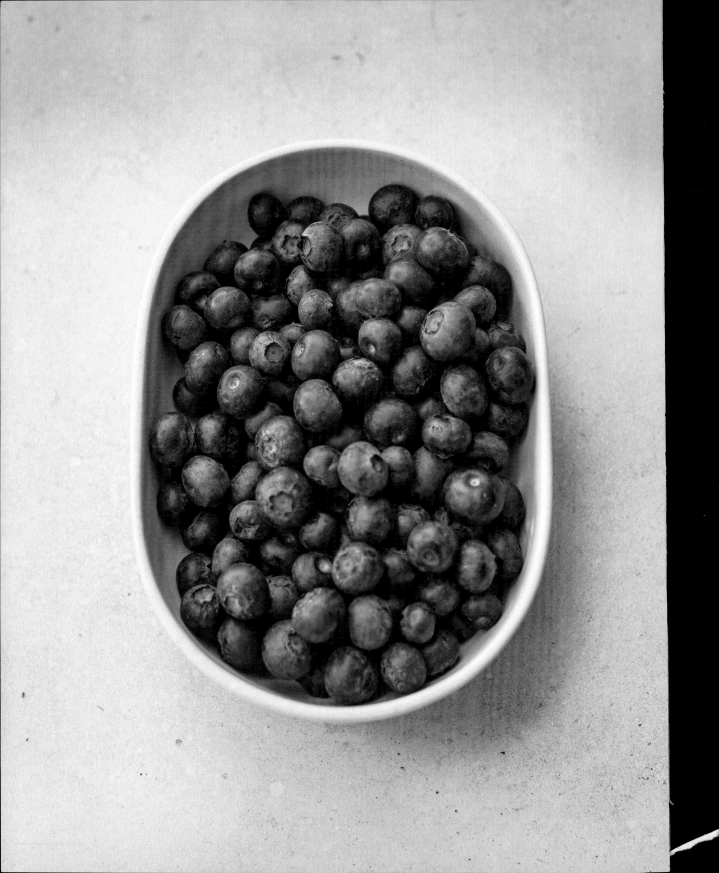

the FastDiet cookbook

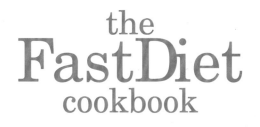

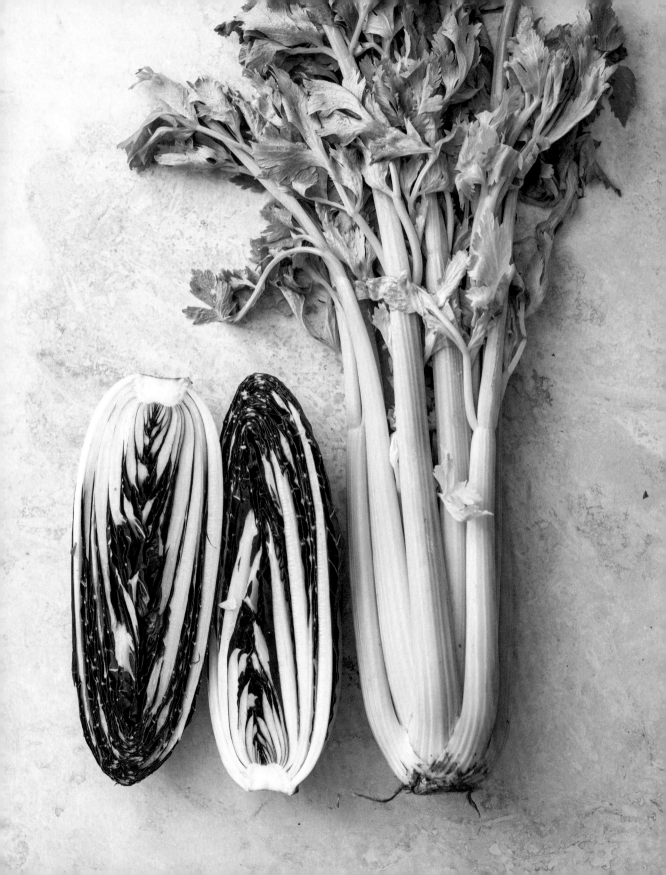

Also by Mimi Spencer

The FastDiet (with Dr. Michael Mosley)

101 Things to Do Before You Diet

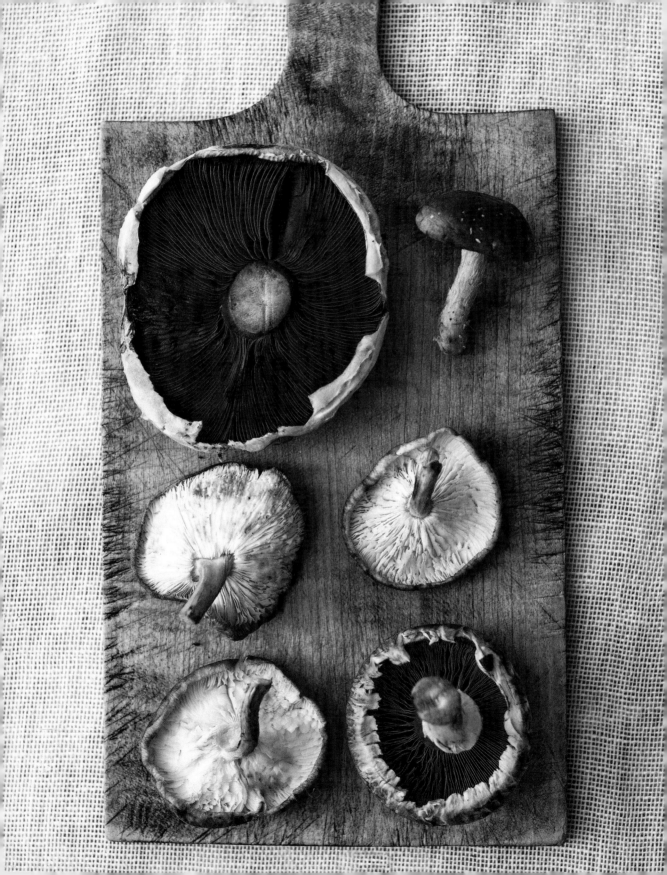

the
FastDiet
cookbook

150 Delicious, Calorie-Controlled Meals

to Make Your Fasting Days Easy

MIMI SPENCER

WITH DR. SARAH SCHENKER

PHOTOGRAPHY BY ROMAS FOORD

ATRIA PAPERBACK

New York   London   Toronto   Sydney   New Delhi

ATRIA PAPERBACK

A Division of Simon & Schuster, Inc.
1230 Avenue of the Americas
New York, NY 10020

Text copyright © 2013 by Mimi Spencer Ltd
Photography copyright © 2013 by Romas Foord
A slightly different version of this work was previously published
as *The Fast Diet Recipe Book* in 2013 in Great Britain by Short Books.

All rights reserved, including the right to reproduce this book or portions
thereof in any form whatsoever. For information, address Atria Books Subsidiary
Rights Department, 1230 Avenue of the Americas, New York, NY 10020.

First Atria Paperback edition July 2013

ATRIA PAPERBACK and colophon are trademarks of Simon & Schuster, Inc.

For information about special discounts for bulk purchases,
please contact Simon & Schuster Special Sales at
1-866-506-1949 or business@simonandschuster.com.

The Simon & Schuster Speakers Bureau can bring authors
to your live event. For more information or to book an event,
contact the Simon & Schuster Speakers Bureau at
1-866-248-3049 or visit our website at www.simonspeakers.com.

Manufactured in the United States of America

10   9   8   7   6   5   4   3   2   1

Library of Congress Cataloging-in-Publication Data is available.

ISBN 978-1-4767-4919-8
ISBN 978-1-4767-4986-0 (pbk)
ISBN 978-1-4767-4920-4 (ebook)

For Debs

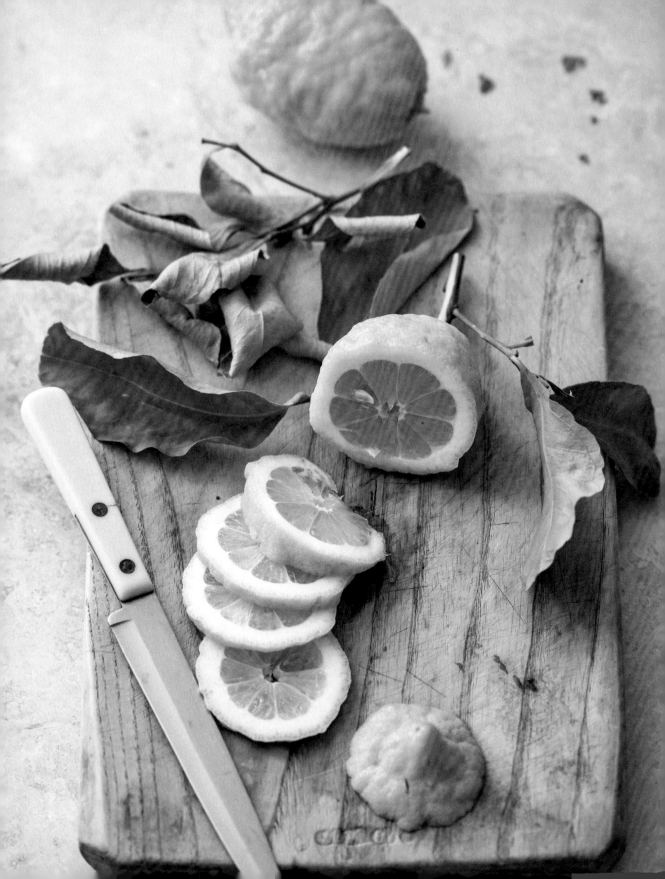

contents

foreword

by Dr. Michael Mosley

When I embarked on my self-experiment into intermittent fasting—back in 2012, while researching a TV documentary—I had little idea quite how great an impact it would have. A year later, and the FastDiet has become a way of life for many people on both sides of the Atlantic and beyond. What started as an examination of the latest research into the health benefits and weight-loss potential of occasional calorie restriction has turned into something real and palpable, something with visible, human consequences. E-mails flood in, like this one from Richard:

"Last year I was wearing size XL shirts; yesterday I tried on a size small shirt while out shopping, and it almost fit, apart from it being too tight around the chest (damn those pecs). This diet is awesome—thanks, Michael, you're quite literally a lifesaver."

When I'm asked why the FastDiet has been so widely embraced, I can offer any number of explanations, but I think the main reason it has struck a chord is because it works. The first couple of weeks can be tough, but once you have adapted to the method, you should find that occasional calorie restriction becomes a positive part of everyday life, always leavened by the knowledge that the next day you can eat as you normally would. You can still bake cakes. You can still eat steak and fries. Just not every day.

The question of "what to eat" while fasting is critical to the feasibility and sustainability of the method. As Mimi writes in this engaging book, the key ingredients for successful fast day food are plants and proteins. Eat the right things on a fast day and you'll enjoy not only nutrient-rich meals, but also a surprisingly large volume of filling food. Better still, with the recipes in this book, you'll be eating delicious, appealing dishes—dishes that you can easily share with friends and family without feeling isolated, fussy, or anchored to impractical and convoluted dieting rules. On your fast days you will be mainly skipping carbs, but nonfasting members of your

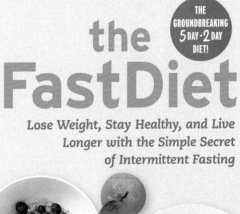

#1 *NEW YORK TIMES* BESTSELLER
DR. MICHAEL MOSLEY and MIMI SPENCER

THE GROUNDBREAKING 5 DAY-2 DAY DIET!

the **FastDiet**

Lose Weight, Stay Healthy, and Live Longer with the Simple Secret of Intermittent Fasting

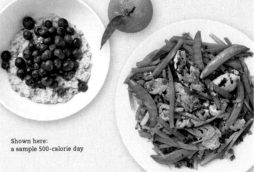

Shown here:
a sample 500-calorie day

family can eat the same food, perhaps topped up with pasta, rice, or potatoes.

Every calorie in this book has been counted by nutritionist Dr. Sarah Schenker, and each dish is carefully balanced to give you the best possible chance of a successful fast day. We hope, of course, that you'll discover that these recipes are so good, you'll want to use them on non–fast days too. Be our guest. As time goes on, you may well find that your taste in food changes, and you gravitate toward healthier, leaner, lighter options on any day of the week. The point is that these recipes will help you eat well and stay healthy, whether you are dieting or not.

This is the next step in the FastDiet story. I feel hugely fortunate to have become involved in something that already feels like it is making a real difference to so many lives.

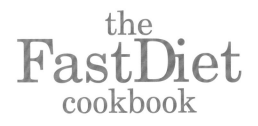

the
FastDiet
cookbook

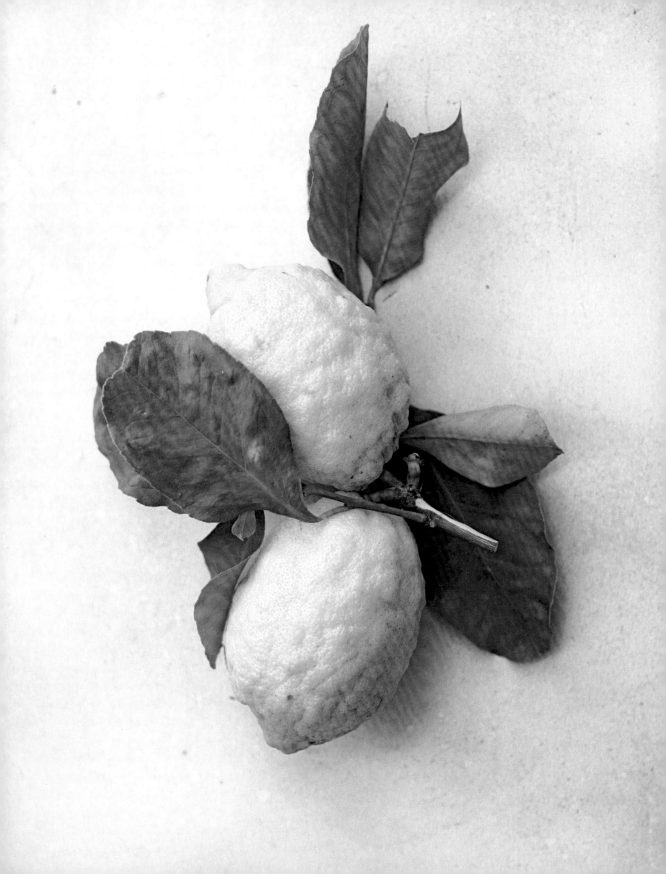

CHAPTER ONE

ALL YOU NEED TO KNOW ABOUT THE FASTDIET

How the FastDiet Went Global

When Dr. Michael Mosley and I started to sketch out plans for *The FastDiet* in October 2012, we had little idea that its impact would prove to be so great. In the months since, the book has received a hugely positive response, and interest around the world is growing daily, in Korea, Brazil, Israel, Australia, Taiwan, the United States— anywhere people are looking for a leaner, fitter life. Hundreds of people have written to us, often with great tenderness and emotion, about their weight loss and health improvements. There has been much enthusiasm from people in the public eye, too. As British food writer and cook Hugh Fearnley-Whittingstall wrote in the newspaper *The Guardian,* "I find myself beguiled, for the first time ever, really, by a new diet. *The FastDiet,* by Michael Mosley and Mimi Spencer, makes a compelling promise that with regular fasting (they propose two days out of every seven) you will quickly lose weight . . . I believe in this fasting thing, I really do . . . I've lost eight pounds already, and I find the whole thing rather exhilarating. I feel I might just be part of a health revolution."

Allison Pearson, a columnist at *The Daily Telegraph,* described *The FastDiet* as her "new bible" and added, "I no longer feel the need to sleep in the afternoon. My stomach has definitely shrunk. The other night it protested when I tried to finish dinner: a world first. Scientists swear that the fasting diet will add years to your life. Me, I'm just happy to have finally shifted that stubborn baby weight. About time, too. The baby was seventeen last week."

At thefastdiet.co.uk, the comments and questions keep rolling in. The FastDiet has always been a conversation, never a set of commandments; we are not interested in promoting diet dependency, only in investigating an idea that appears to have significant health-giving potential. So we're fascinated by your stories, your successes, and your occasional blips, and as the science develops, we hope to have more answers to share.

In the meantime, many of you have requested inspiration for what to eat on your twice-weekly fast days. If you'll excuse the obvious oxymoron, *The FastDiet Cookbook* is our answer. But before we pull on an apron and raid the fridge, it's worth taking a brief detour into the science behind intermittent fasting, and how the FastDiet came to be.

In the Beginning . . .

In 2012, Dr. Michael Mosley, an overweight medically trained journalist, discovered that he was a borderline diabetic with very high levels of "bad" cholesterol. He was told by his doctor that he needed to start medication and that unless he did something about it, within ten years he would be swallowing eight pills a day, like the average sixty-year-old European or American.

Keen to find a nonpharmaceutical way to change his fate, he tracked down and interviewed scientists doing cutting-edge research into intermittent fasting. "Fasting," in this context, does not mean avoiding all food; it simply means cutting back, for relatively short periods of time, on some foods.

In our society, we tend to eat all the time— and that constant overeating doesn't just make us fat; it also keeps our bodies in permanent

1

"go" mode. This leads to elevated levels of hormones like insulin and IGF-1 (insulin-like growth factor 1), which cause metabolic changes in the body. While this is a perfectly normal response to eating, the problem comes when these hormones dominate all the time; this can bring an increased risk of developing a range of diseases including diabetes, heart disease, and some cancers.

Cutting back on calories, by contrast, reduces insulin levels and gives your system a chance to rid itself of old and worn-out cells—a bit like taking your car into the garage for an occasional tune-up; doing so will almost certainly ensure that it goes on running in peak condition for longer.

The Importance of Fat Loss Versus Weight Loss

Weight is, of course, easy to measure—you just need a bathroom scale. But what people sometimes forget in their obsession with losing weight is that what they really want to lose is fat.

Not all fat, however, is equally bad. Fat on the thighs and buttocks, for example, appears to be less of a health risk than excess belly fat, known as visceral fat. Visceral fat significantly increases the risk of heart disease and diabetes, which is why you should aim to have a waist (as measured around your belly button) that is less than half your height.

While losing fat, you want to preserve as much muscle as possible. One reason this is important is that muscle is metabolically active; in other words, if you take two people who are the same weight, but one is muscular and the other fat, the muscular one not only is likely to be healthier but also will burn more calories, even when sleeping. People with more muscle have a better chance of keeping weight off.

You can help preserve muscle by maintaining—or better still, increasing—the amount you exercise. This could simply mean walking more and always taking the stairs, or performing more vigorous activities such as weight training. As an added bonus, studies have shown that you are likely to burn more fat if you exercise in the fasted state rather than in the fed state.[1]

Intermittent Fasting and Fat Loss

One of the great problems with crash diets or yo-yo dieting is that although some of the weight you lose will be fat, much of it will be muscle: On a conventional diet you will lose about 75 percent of the weight as fat and 25 percent as muscle. When you regain the weight, as most people inevitably do, the weight you regain is almost all fat.

The human trials that have been done so far suggest that intermittent fasting is unusual in that the weight loss appears to be almost all fat, and, importantly, much of the fat you lose is the dangerous type from around the gut.

A number of studies involving overweight volunteers doing ADF (alternate-day fasting)[2] found that when individuals were asked to eat a quarter of their normal calories one day, then eat whatever they liked the next, they lost significant amounts of weight and saw substantial improvements in their cholesterol and blood sugars. A surprising finding was that when allowed to feast, people did not do so. They reported not feeling particularly hungry after a fast day and rarely ate more than 110 percent of their normal calories. This is borne out by anecdotal evidence, too: Many people on the FastDiet simply don't feel ravenous the following day. Their appetite and attitudes toward food seem to change, and healthier eating seems to become part of their everyday life.

Another surprising finding was that on this form of IF, individuals lost more body fat than expected. In the most recent study of thirty-two volunteers followed for three months, the average weight loss was nearly 9 pounds, almost all fat, and they lost an average of 3 inches around the waist.

In another study, 107 women were randomly allocated either to a diet where they cut their food intake to 650 calories for two days a week and tried to stick to a healthy diet for the rest of the week, or to a diet where they consumed the same total number of calories, but spread out over the week.[3]

After six months, the two-day fasters had lost an average of 13¼ pounds of fat and 3 inches from their waists, compared with 10¾ pounds and 2 inches for the daily dieters. They also had much greater improvements in their cholesterol and insulin levels.

Enter the FastDiet

So there is evidence, from human trials, of success with different forms of intermittent fasting. After some self-experimenting, Michael settled for a form he called 5:2, which is the basis of the FastDiet.

The rules are very simple.

- You eat normally for five days a week, but for two days a week you eat one-quarter of your normal calorie intake—about 600 calories for men, 500 for women.

- You can do your fast days back to back or split them. Michael tried both ways and found he preferred to split them. He did his fast days on Mondays and Thursdays.

- He also split his 600-calorie allowance on those days into breakfast and an evening meal.

On this regimen, Michael lost 19 pounds of body fat and his blood markers improved beyond

recognition. He found that once he had lost the fat, he could keep it off (normally the hard bit) by using a 6:1 method of cutting calories to a quarter of his normal intake just once a week and by always taking the stairs.

Commissioned to write about intermittent fasting for *The Times* (London), I soon followed Michael's lead and in four months lost 20 pounds, returning to my "wedding weight" at the age of 45. Toward the end of 2012, inspired by the success of the 5:2 pattern, Michael and I cowrote *The FastDiet*. It became an instant best seller on both sides of the Atlantic. Intermittent fasting really is, as Hugh Fearnley-Whittingstall says, starting to look like a "health revolution."

We believe that the FastDiet's success has to do with its flexibility, its simple basic tenets, and the fact that it is backed by solid science. From a psychological point of view, its indisputable attraction is that calorie restriction is limited to only two days a week, leaving the rest of the time blissfully free of worry.

So Where's the Catch?

There are some people for whom intermittent fasting is not recommended; however, there is no evidence of significant side effects. Some people may experience headaches or constipation, particularly at first; these can generally be alleviated by drinking lots of calorie-free fluids and eating foods that are rich in fiber. Some find they get hungry late at night and can't sleep well. It should help if you have a more substantial evening meal, or perhaps a glass of milk before bedtime.

In some ways, the FastDiet is simply a modern take on an ancient idea. In one form or another, fasting has been practiced for centuries by most of the great religions, and if done properly seems to be extremely safe.

There are, however, a number of myths around eating that might dissuade you from trying intermittent fasting. These include the ideas that

- You need to eat whenever you feel hungry.

- Eating every few hours will increase your metabolic rate.

- If you don't eat every few hours, your blood sugar will fall and you will feel faint.

None of these widely held beliefs is backed by science. Certainly, fasting in any form can be tough to start with, but you should discover that short bouts of hunger are manageable and soon pass. Similarly, there is no metabolic advantage to spreading your calories over the day, nor is there any evidence that short periods without food will cause your blood sugar to plunge to seriously low levels. Most nights, you go 12 hours without eating anyway, and many people feel fine with a late breakfast.

You may want to get medical support before you start or if you have any questions. You will find a wealth of tips and supportive advice from those who have already tried it at thefastdiet .co.uk, where you can also contribute your experiences. By now, though, you're probably feeling hungry. Time to move out of the classroom and into the kitchen.

Do You Really Want to Cook on a Fast Day?

We're all different. When fasting, you may not wish to spend time in the kitchen, surrounded by ingredients and temptation. Some people want speed and simplicity, preferring to eat sparingly and basically—and there are plenty of ideas in this book that will be useful to people who want to eat in this way.

Others, like me, prefer to make fast day food interesting and flavorful, with fresh, low-

calorie meals to bookend the day. I can't promise the glorious depth of glossy butter sauces or the caramelized toffee you may find in other cookbooks. But I can offer wholesome, well-balanced, nutritious, engaging, pretty, fresh food that's simple to prepare and easy to understand. I also suggest more unusual dishes to stretch the imagination and take us all on a bit of a journey.

A Diet for Foodies

In fact, I would even argue that the FastDiet is a "diet for foodies." While you restrict calories—deliciously, if you wish, and with as much fanfare as you dare within the calorie budget—on two days each week, on the other five days you can eat absolutely normally. We don't suggest bingeing, but we do advise forgetting that you are on a diet at all. Five days a week, the FastDiet is—and should be—an irrelevance.

What intermittent fasting *will* do, however, is encourage you to cut back on processed foods, together with their attendant preservatives and packaging. It insists that you eat fresh, good produce for two days a week. The upshot over time? We are all more engaged with the food on our plates.

. . . and the Frugal . . .

On the FastDiet, you occasionally eat less, and therefore you spend less, an idea well suited to these days of austerity. One FastDiet fan named Snorvey writes of his shopping bills: "They're certainly lower. I hadn't even thought about it till someone mentioned it elsewhere, but at a rough guestimate, they're about 15 percent lower. A projected amount of 395,000 calories of food not eaten per year (between two of us—the wife is following the 5:2 as well) would add up to a fair bit of money over the year."

. . . and Non-Fasters, too

This book will help you develop a loose repertoire of meals that are sometimes hasty, always tasty, but above all low in fast-release carbs, which means that if you are calorie counting in the traditional way—day in, day out—this book will serve you equally well; you could happily use it as an everyday low-cal cookbook.

In fact, one of the key changes that will hopefully occur over the course of several months on the FastDiet, as many fasting fans have attested, is that your appetite will alter and you will start to crave the good things in life *on any day:* You may develop a yen for fresh salads, fabulous soups, lean proteins, good carbs, sparky flavor combinations, or satiating breakfasts that don't unduly bother the frying pan. You'll find many recipes here that meet these requirements. The book works, too, for people who are dairy- or wheat-intolerant, as very few of the recipes contain either. And it's also pretty good for vegetarians, as lots of the recipes rely on plant proteins.

When you're not fasting, the book still has plenty to offer. Play around with some of the ingredients, bump up the numbers, add a chunk of sourdough bread or a tumble of noodles, rice on the side or buttered corn on the cob . . . all of them will make for good eating any day of the week.

CHAPTER TWO

WHAT, WHEN, AND HOW TO EAT ON A FAST DAY

What to Eat?

There are very few rules here. No weighing out matchbox-size portions of cheese. No measuring, fretting, or complicated equations. In a nutshell, the fast day meal mantra is: *mostly plants and protein.*

This is the basis of all of the recipes in this book. Okay, there's a little fat, too, a few slow-burn carbs, perhaps a drop of dairy. But "mostly p&p" pretty much sums it up. The only other word we'd add is *variety*. A varied plate of food promises a diverse lineup of nutrients and will add interest to your day.

So what should be on your fast day plate?

FIRST, THE QUESTION OF CARBS

One of the more important hormones determining your health is insulin. When you eat, particularly foods rich in carbohydrates, your blood sugar levels rise, and in response the pancreas churns out insulin. Insulin helps remove glucose from your blood and store it in your liver or muscles as glycogen. Insulin also stops your body from using fat as a fuel.

If you constantly eat lots of sugary, carbohydrate-rich foods (and drinks), your body copes by producing increasing amounts of insulin. In time, your cells become less responsive, and your body becomes caught in a vicious circle where it has to produce ever-higher levels of insulin to get the same result. This can lead to type 2 diabetes, which in turn significantly increases your risk of heart attack, stroke, impotence, blindness, and losing your extremities due to poor circulation. It is also associated with brain shrinkage and dementia.

An added problem is that as well as being a sugar and fat controller, insulin and a related hormone called IGF-1 (insulin-like growth factor 1) stimulate the growth and turnover of new cells. This constant activity increases the risk that some of these cells will turn cancerous. High levels of insulin and IGF-1 are associated with a range of cancers including breast, bowel, and prostate cancer.

There is good evidence that restricting your calorie intake, and in particular your carbohydrate intake, for a couple of days a week will improve insulin sensitivity and cut levels of circulating insulin. The recipes in this book are based on that approach, referencing the glycemic index (GI) and glycemic load (GL) of the ingredients. You'll recall that the GI rating measures the effect of a food on blood sugar relative to pure glucose (which scores 100). The GL takes into account how much carbohydrate is in a food. Watermelon, for example, has a high GI but a relatively low GL, as it's mostly water.

On the days when you are fasting, you still eat, but you should aim to eat foods with a low glycemic index; in other words, foods that do not cause spikes in blood sugar. Most vegetables are a FastDieter's friend because they have a low GI, and also because they provide a lot of bulk for very few calories, keeping hunger at bay.

PROTEIN

Unlike fast-release carbohydrates, protein keeps you feeling full for longer, which is one reason to have plenty of it in fast day meals.

When people see the word *protein* they generally think of meat. Though chicken and beef are rich in protein, there is also protein in fish, milk, nuts, seeds, and legumes. Proteins are essential nutrients, the building blocks of your body tissue as well as a major fuel source. Unlike fat or carbohydrates, protein is not stored by your body; instead, food containing protein is broken down by your digestive system to provide amino acids, which are then used for a whole range of vital activities, from building muscle to creating hormones, enzymes, and neurotransmitters.

Because your body does not store protein, we recommend that you boost the protein content of your diet on fast days so that it becomes a greater proportion of your daily diet *on just those days*. That way, you benefit from its satiating effects (protein really does make you feel fuller for longer than carbs) and you will have adequate levels of protein at all times. On nonfasting days, of course, we recommend that you eat as usual and don't concern yourself with dieting.

The recommended daily level for protein is roughly 55 grams. If you want to be more precise, one guideline suggests 0.83 gram per kilogram (2.2 pounds) of body weight, which for a 154-pound (70-kilogram) man works out to about 58 grams a day, and for a 132-pound (60-kilogram) woman, to about 50 grams.

PLANTS

The pigments that plants produce don't simply attract pollinating insects; they represent some of the thousands of bioactive compounds, known as phytochemicals, that keep plants alive and healthy. By eating a wide range of different-colored plants, we also get those benefits, and on a fast day, they are the central event.

Green
"Leafy greens," which include spinach, chard, lettuce, and kale, are a good source of minerals such as magnesium, manganese, and potassium. Another class of green vegetables, the cruciferous ones, are those that contain sulfur and organosulfur compounds. These include cabbage, cauliflower, broccoli, and other members of the Brassica family. Sulfur is essential for the production of glutathione, an important antioxidant, as well as amino acids such as methionine and taurine.

Different vegetables will bring different things to your plate. Spinach, for example, contains lots of calcium, but not in a form that the body can readily absorb; if you want calcium, you are better off with broccoli. You can learn more from the Nutritional Bonus (NB) included with most recipes in this book.

Orange and Yellow
Flavonoid comes from the Latin word *flavus*, meaning yellow, and in a plant this substance attracts insects for pollination and protects against harmful ultraviolet light. In humans there is some evidence that eating flavonoids helps combat the risks of allergy, inflammation, and infection.[1] Fruits and vegetables with a significant amount of yellow or orange, such as carrots, melons, tomatoes, peppers, and squash, contain a particular type of flavonoid called carotenoid. The type of carotenoid in carrots can be converted to retinol, an active form of vitamin A, important for healthy eyesight, bone growth, and regulation of the immune system.

Red
There are a huge number of carotenoids with different properties. One other class, called lycopene, produces the color red. You'll find lots of lycopene in tomatoes. It is an antioxidant and a recent study showed it helps reduce the risk of having a stroke.[2] Oddly enough, cooking tomatoes boosts the levels of lycopene, because heat helps break down the plant's thick cell walls, making the nutrient more available for absorption.[3] Unfortunately, heat also destroys vitamin C, so it's a trade-off.

Blue and purple

Blue and purple foods get their color from a group of flavonoids called anthocyanins. You'll find decent levels in blackberries, blueberries, purple carrots, and red cabbage. There is some evidence that anthocyanin-rich blueberries may slow the rate at which memory and cognitive function decline as people age.[4]

White

Examples include garlic, white onions, shallots, and leeks, all rich in allyl sulfur compounds. Although there is no compelling proof that garlic will ward off vampires, it does appear to be quite good at killing microorganisms; traditionally, it has been eaten raw to treat coughs, colds, and croup.

VEGETABLES: THE RAW AND THE COOKED

There is debate about the best way to cook vegetables in order to retain as much of their goodness as possible. The answer is . . . there is no single answer. It all depends.

The reason we cook food is to make it more digestible; cooking tenderizes meat and breaks down tough vegetable fiber, something our digestive systems can no longer really cope with. But cooking also affects certain vitamins. Vitamin C, for example, is fragile and easily lost when heated, whereas lycopene is enhanced by the cooking process. If you live on a raw food diet, it's likely that you will enjoy high levels of vitamin C but low levels of lycopene. Boiling and steaming carrots, spinach, and cabbage will also increase the bioavailability of carotene while reducing some other vitamin content. Our advice would be to mix up the raw and the cooked. Have both. Often.

Why vegetables beat fruit every time

When people are told they need to eat more fruit and vegetables, they frequently respond by simply eating more fruit. On the face of it, that's not a bad thing as fruits, like vegetables, are packed with nutritional goodies. Unfortunately, many fruits are also packed with calories and fructose. Vegetables, by contrast, provide a lot of bulk and masses of fiber and have limited impact on your blood sugars and therefore on your insulin.

Some fruits, like strawberries and blueberries, have surprisingly few calories and do not adversely affect your blood sugar (unless, of course, you drench them in sugar), which is why you will find them in the recipes here. Black currants and raspberries do respectably well, too. Others, however, such as pineapple, are high in sugars. A large banana, for example, has about 120 calories, while a large carrot has more like 30 calories and a large serving of broccoli about the same. So while we would certainly encourage people to eat fruit, on fast days we recommend that sweet-tasting fruit be rationed.

If you do choose to eat fruit, make it fresh, not dried, as the drying process concentrates calories. A 3½-ounce (100-gram) serving of fresh apricots, for instance, typically has about 31 calories while the same quantity of dried apricots clocks in at four times the calorie cost.

To juice or not to juice

Although fruit is generally a nutritious option, juice is ultimately a higher-sugar, lower-nutrient version of its source. Juicing inevitably reduces or eliminates fruit and vegetable skin—yet those vital health-giving pigments, the seats of flavonoids and carotenoids, are concentrated in the skin and, in some cases, the pulp. Another case of your grandmother being right: eat the skin.

Plant skins are also the primary, if not the sole, source of fiber, important for the health of your gut—and also for slowing down the digestion and absorption of sugars. The take-home message is this: Juice can offer a decent source of nutrients on days when it's hard to work in your usual amount of fruit and vegetables, but it's not an adequate substitute for the real, whole source.

GOOD FATS AND WHY YOU NEED THEM

Fat matters, and there *is* such a thing as too little fat in the diet. This is because certain vitamins (A, D, E, and K) are fat soluble, which means that they require fat in order to be absorbed by the body (B vitamins and vitamin C are water soluble and don't need fat for absorption). Essentially, dietary fat ferries vitamins across the cell walls of the small intestine, into the bloodstream, and on to the liver, where they are stored till the body needs them. But not all fats are equal. On a fast day, reduce saturated fats (animal fats), avoid trans fats, and instead choose plant fats from nuts, seeds, olives, or avocados. You need only a little, added to a vitamin-rich meal. The recipes in this book provide just that, so you don't even have to do the math.

WHY SOUP?

You'll notice that there are plenty of recipes for soup here, and you may question their inclusion,

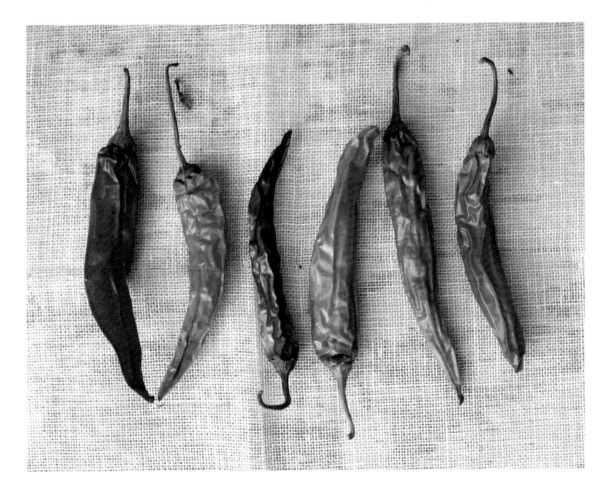

given our advice on juicing fruit. Soups are a special case, and well worth including on a fast day menu. Research has shown that, while fluids generally have lower satiety value than solid foods, soups break the rule: They are brilliantly satiating, leading to what scientists at Purdue University call "reductions of hunger and increases of fullness . . . comparable to the solid foods."[5] In short, soup gets you full and keeps you there. Great news for a fast day. Better yet, a homemade soup uses up elderly vegetables from the fridge, never tastes the same twice, and will warm the cockles of your heart.

When to Eat?

The timetable is largely your own. Eat when it suits you, your family, your lifestyle, your day. The recipes here are divided into breakfasts and suppers, but there's no definitive reason to eat them at those times, other than that they mark a traditional start and end to a day. Many of these recipes work well as anytime meals, to suit the pattern that you have developed. You may wish to skip breakfast or dodge dinner. That it is entirely up to you. The FastDiet has been called the ultimate flexible diet with good reason.

It is, however, important to aim for as long a fasting window between bouts of eating as possible—this is where many of the health benefits of intermittent fasting lie, as readers of our first book will already know. On a fast day, Michael and I both have breakfast at 7:00 a.m. and supper at 7:00 p.m., giving us an ideal twelve-hour window. You may opt for something different. We are not dispensing rules, simply offering suggestions.

It's worth revisiting these words from *The FastDiet*: "Your aim is to carve out a food-free breathing space for your body. Going to 510 calories (or 615 for a man) won't hurt—it won't obliterate a fast. Indeed, the idea of slashing calories to a quarter of your daily intake on a fast day is simply one that has been clinically proven to have systemic effects on the metabolism. While there's no particular 'magic' to 500 or 600 calories, do try to stick to these numbers; you need clear parameters to make the strategy effective in the medium term."

But the crucial thing is to find a way that works for you. Which means you may need to cope with feeling a little . . .

HUNGRY?

As many successful fasters now know, hunger is not the beast we imagine it to be; it is generally manageable and usually fairly modest, and the pangs soon pass. Of course, the whole idea of the FastDiet is to give your body an occasional break from eating, periods of "downtime" when it does not have to process food. Some people will find, after trying it for a few weeks, that they can comfortably go up to 12 hours without food. For others this will prove too challenging. The most important thing, remember, is finding a system that you can stick to.

That is why this book does suggest suitable snacks for your fast days (see Chapter 13). If you must snack, do it with awareness and frugality, avoid carbs, and always keep an eye on the GI. Remember, too, that any snacking will eat into your allotted calories—you will be eating the same number of calories, but they'll be spread out over the course of the day. Does this undermine the benefits of intermittent fasting? We just don't know; the studies have not been done. The important thing, in our view, is to not be put off or to give up at the first hurdle because you find the experience of fasting too difficult. If snacking helps you to start with, that is fine.

Of course, if you eat the right things on a fast day, it's possible that you'll escape hunger entirely. Time, then, to introduce the recipes and how the book works.

CHAPTER THREE

THE NUTS AND BOLTS OF THE BOOK

Some of the recipes are gloriously simple, others are more complex; some are favorites adapted for the FastDiet, while others introduce new flavor combinations. Some will get you walking or gardening. Others will send you to the cupboard for a bunch of cans.

- The book includes both simple recipes and leisurely recipes, allowing you to spend as much or as little time as you please preparing your fast day food.

- Each recipe has a clear calorie count per portion, with calorie contents increasing as you go through each chapter. The idea is that you can choose a breakfast and a supper, in whatever combination you wish, to arrive at your 500- or 600-calorie budget for the day. For good pairings, refer to the examples in the Meal Plans.

- Some recipes serve two or more—simply because the cooking method works better that way (it's difficult to make a sauce work for one)—but the calorie count is always for a single portion.

- Feel free to bump up the leafy vegetables in most of the recipes; it won't make much difference to overall calorie intake, but will add bulk and welcome nutrients.

- Each recipe clearly shows its Nutritional Bonus (look for NB), together with the GI or GL score where useful.

Finding Flavor Without Fat

We all know that adding a generous slab of butter to almost anything will make it taste fantastic. Our job here is to fill the flavor vacuum with something other than saturated fat. In this race, the humble lemon is in pole position: Lemon juice is a remarkable flavor enhancer, capable of lending goodness to countless slow-cooked savory dishes. Roasted garlic is similarly delicious. You'll discover that plenty of the recipes in this book depend on the "fantastic five"—lime juice, soy sauce, fresh ginger, garlic, and Asian fish sauce—which deliver mighty bursts of flavor with the merest suggestion of calories. Herbs and spices also feature heavily in fast day cooking. Cumin seeds, cardamom pods, sweet Spanish paprika, dense green basil, delicate tendrils of dill . . . they are not garnishes here, but central to the proceedings. Chiles, too, are worth their weight in gold. Do remember to wear gloves when you slice or chop them—your eyes will thank you later.

Here, then, are the basic ingredients for a fast day cupboard.

CARBS

For an alternative to pasta or wheat noodles, try shirataki noodles. Made from a water-soluble, plant-based fiber called glucomannan, they have no fat, sugar, gluten, or starch. No flavor either, so call upon the fantastic five. If you need a bread substitute, have a thin rye crispbread. But as a rule, avoid white carbs on a fast day.

GRAINS

Though carbs are necessarily limited on a fast day, those you do eat should be whole grains, not refined ones—they have more fiber, B vitamins, and other nutrients, and take longer to digest. Quinoa is a great source of protein, as is bulgur, while the best fast day rice is brown basmati. Old-fashioned oatmeal outranks the rest: less processed, more bulky.

LEGUMES

Legumes such as lentils, chickpeas, split peas, and a whole world of beans are excellent sources of plant protein and fiber, and rank low on the GI scale. Toss cans of pintos, borlotti, or butter beans (experiment—you can't really go wrong) into your shopping cart—you'll find plenty of recipes here to turn a can into a dinner.

CANNED GOODS

You won't get far around here without a can of diced tomatoes, so always have one or two on hand (plus a tube of tomato paste to add bass-note depth to all manner of savory dishes). I particularly like fire-roasted tomatoes, which are especially tasty. A couple of cans of tuna (in spring water to minimize calories) and a jar or can of anchovy fillets? Vital.

FATS

Choose "smart fats" over saturated fats, which means butter must take a backseat. Instead, use

Olive oil A monounsaturated oil that is more resistant to the damaging effects of heat than polyunsaturated oils such as corn oil. A recent study from the University of Munich found that olive oil keeps you feeling fuller longer.[1] You need expensive extra virgin olive oil only for salad dressings and drizzling; use standard olive oil for cooking.

Unrefined flaxseed oil Flaxseeds are rich in alpha linolenic acid (an omega-3 fat) and are a condensed source of antiviral, antioxidant lignans. Use cold-pressed flaxseed oil for salad dressings (don't cook with it or you'll annihilate the goodness).

Coconut oil Slower to oxidize and less damaged by heat than other cooking oils; a good source of heart-healthy fatty acids, and it shouldn't your raise cholesterol.

Canola oil Only 7 percent saturated fat (butter is 51 percent), and unlike olive oil, it doesn't degrade at high heat, so this is one for the wok.

DAIRY

Steer clear of heavy dairy on a fast day. Some recipes in this book call for crème fraîche or unflavored low-fat yogurt. It's worth noting that certain cheeses are lower in calories than others: Feta, for example, is made from sheep's milk and is a good source of protein, calcium, and vitamin B_{12}. Low-fat mozzarella is a handy staple in the fridge.

SEEDS AND NUTS

Sunflower and pumpkin seeds are nutritious additions to morning muesli and salad suppers, bringing good plant fats to your diet.

Nuts are satiating, full of fiber, and handy to have around when hunger calls. Though they are generally calorific, it's worth keeping packets of pine nuts, almonds, pistachios, and walnuts (rich in omega-9s) to add to salads and oatmeal.

FLAVORINGS

Your own tastes will dictate exactly what you keep on this shelf (in the cupboard and in the fridge).

Bouillon cubes and powders, including Vegeta
As many spices as you can usefully own without anyone complaining
Red pepper flakes, cayenne pepper, and smoked paprika
Tabasco and Worcestershire sauces
Garlic, lots of it, preferably fresh, but also pureed or chopped (in a jar) to keep in the fridge
Fresh ginger to slice into pretty much anything, from stir-fries to tea
Mustard of any and all varieties; they do different jobs: spiky yellow English; ochre, rounded Dijon; grainy Dijon for mellow bite and texture
Onions, shallots, green onions or scallions—the last gives you onion flavor with minimum fuss
Asian fish sauce, soy sauce (choose a low-sodium version), and mirin
White wine vinegar, red wine vinegar, cider vinegar, and rice vinegar: like mustard, vinegars have subtly different roles to play
Canned diced green chiles, for days when you can't be bothered to chop

Sweeteners
Avoid refined sugar on a fast day. Honey, though natural, will spike your blood sugar. Rather than using lab-developed sugar substitutes, try adding a sprinkling of coconut to breakfast porridge, or use a touch of raw agave nectar: known in Mexico as *aguamiel*, or "honey water," agave is a low-GI sweetener produced from a cactus-like plant.

Salt and Pepper
I would always use glittering coarse sea salt or flaky salt, and peppercorns to grind fresh in a grinder, all of which have a glorious fragrance and texture.

Ten Things Slim People Keep in the Fridge

1. Lemons

2. Free-range eggs

3. Reduced-fat hummus

4. Nonstarchy vegetables (cauliflower, broccoli, peppers, radishes, cherry tomatoes, celery, cucumber, mushrooms, lettuce, sugar snaps, snow peas, and a bag of young spinach)

5. Feta, cottage cheese, and low-fat mozzarella

6. Sprouts (alfalfa, mung, soy, and all their friends)

7. Pickled guindillas, jalapeños, and cornichons (or small dill pickles)

8. Fresh strawberries

9. Fresh chiles

10. Unflavored low-fat yogurt

And in the Freezer . . .

1. Ginger; easier to grate from the frozen root

2. Sofritto, aka mirepoix (finely diced onion, carrot, and celery in a 2:1:1 ratio), to save time and energy when cooking any number of recipes

3. Homemade vegetable, chicken, and fish stock, frozen in ice cube trays and transferred to heavy-duty plastic bags, and in 1- and 2-cup plastic containers

4. Fresh herbs, frozen with a little water in ice cube trays

5. Soups: double the recipe and freeze for another day. Thick soups freeze best; you may want to loosen with more stock once thawed.

6. Frozen peas, edamame, and fava beans. Toss them into soups, stews, and (after blanching) salads

7. Frozen blueberries, for a cool little snack (strawberries do not freeze well without added sugar)

The Fast Day Kitchen, Equipped

The recipes here require little expertise and even less equipment. You may, however, find it handy to have the following stashed somewhere in the kitchen.

- Stick blender or canister blender for pureeing

- Food processor

- Multilevel steamer (bamboo or stainless steel), a saucepan with a steamer insert, or a steamer basket

- A mandoline or julienne peeler for shredding vegetables

- Mortar and pestle or mini food processor for grinding spices

- A cast-iron grill pan, to allow fat to run off meat

- Nonstick cookware, including a nonstick wok and nonstick foil (such as Release) to reduce the need for oil

- Silicone brush for oiling

- Parchment paper for lining pans and for steaming foods "en papillote"

- A zester and/or a grater, such as a Microplane

- A kitchen scale; many of the recipes here call for you to weigh ingredients. Don't worry; it's easy and you'll soon get the hang of it.

How to Cook Fast: Tips, Swaps, and Shortcuts

OILS AND FATS

- Whichever cooking oil you choose (see page 12 for your best options), a spray will reduce your use. Some brands of olive oil spray, for example, have less than 1 calorie per spray.

- Alternatively, use a silicone brush to apply oil to the pan and dab away excess with a paper towel.

- To stop ingredients from sticking, add a little water to the pan rather than a slug of oil.

EGGS

- Boiling or poaching means you are not adding any fast day calories.

- A perfectly poached egg has a lovely rounded shape, a soft yet firm white, and a deliciously runny yolk. A good trick to achieve poached perfection is to place the whole (very fresh) egg, in its shell, in boiling water for 15 seconds prior to breaking and poaching as normal.

- Time is, of course, of the essence when it comes to poaching eggs—though you can poach them up to a day in advance. Simply slip the cooked eggs into a bowl of cold water, cover, and refrigerate. To reheat, drain, cover with boiling water, and leave for 2 to 3 minutes, draining well on paper towels.

MEAT

- Cooking poultry with its skin on will maximize flavor and prevent drying out, but don't eat the skin. Much of the fat lies there.

- Roast on a rack over a baking pan to allow excess fat to drip away.

- Similarly, a cast-iron grill pan channels fat into the grooves and away from your plate— as a bonus, you also get a tasty grill-mark effect.

- Whenever possible, cook meat and fish on a barbecue—it's your fat-free summer standby.

- Replace ground beef with mushrooms, textured vegetable protein (TVP), or Quorn to lessen your calorie cost.

- If you do eat beef or lamb, choose grass-fed or pasture-raised meat. It has less fat and more omega-3s than grain-fed meat (and grass or pasture feeding also implies that the animal was humanely raised).

- Extend your meat choices to include lean game. Venison, for example, has a fraction of the fat found in beef.

VEGETABLES

- Scrub vegetables rather than peel them, as many nutrients are found close to the skin. Eating the skins will add fiber to your diet (see page 8).

- Steam vegetables instead of boiling them, or use the microwave; that way their nutrients are more likely to remain intact.

- If you do boil vegetables, use as little water as possible and do not overcook them. Overcooking degrades their flavor and nutritional benefit.

- When browning and caramelizing vegetables, put them in a hot dry pan, then spray with oil, rather than putting the oil in the pan first. This will reduce the amount of oil absorbed during cooking.

- To skin tomatoes, cut an X in the bottom, dunk in boiling water for 30 seconds, cool briefly in ice water, and peel with a sharp knife or a thumbnail.

- To peel garlic, bash the clove with the heel of your hand or immerse first in warm water for 30 seconds.

- To skin roasted peppers, place the blackened peppers in a bowl, cover with plastic wrap for 10 minutes, then peel.

- Don't salt lentils during cooking; it will toughen them. Season when ready to serve.

- As a rule, use fresh herbs rather than dried, as they tend to have more flavor and nutrients. Grow them on a windowsill, or keep cut herbs in jars of water in the fridge like bouquets. Alternatively, wrap fresh herbs in just-damp paper towels and keep them in the crisper.

STOCK

- A good stock is the foundation of countless savory dishes. You can buy ready-made stock in boxes and cans, but making your own is good for the belly and, it has to be said, good for the soul.

- Have stock handy in the freezer; simply heat it

up and add frozen vegetables or herbs, warm through, and you've got yourself a bowl of fast day flavor.

- Roasting bones before adding them to the stockpot will boost color and flavor; a roasted chicken carcass is ideal.

- Don't chuck lone bones: freeze them and make a stock when you have a decent pile.

- Add a bouquet of herbs for more flavor; make your own by tying a bunch of garden herbs with string, making them easy to fish out when they've done their work.

- Adding a teaspoon of vinegar to a stock will aid the extraction of minerals without unduly influencing the flavor.

- Simmer slowly—a good stock should not be rushed—and top up with water to ensure the pot doesn't boil dry.

- Skim off any fat and froth that rise to the top of the pot. Place paper towels on the surface to absorb fat, or chill first to make skimming easier. If keeping stock for later use, retain the layer of fat on top to protect it in the fridge. Simply skim when you're ready to use.

SOUP

- Thicken soup with legumes instead of potatoes. A handful of lentils will do the trick.

- Gravitate toward clear vegetable broths. Miso soup and pho are lower in calories than dense chowders, bisques, and cream soups.

- Vegetable stock generally has a lower fat content than chicken stock.

- If it suits the recipe, leave vegetables whole or in large chunks, rather than pureeing them.

- Make soup in generous batches and freeze; smooth, thick soups perform best. And remember that soups, like stews, often taste better the next day.

- Add miso or bouillon cubes or powder to intensify taste.

- When making a soup base, don't sweat vegetables in butter; use water or a spray of oil.

- If you're not adding fat, you do need to add flavor. Red pepper flakes, cumin, star anise, cloves, a squeeze of lemon, handfuls of herbs—these will all make your soup bowl sing.

- A pinch of sugar will bring out the flavor in tomato-based soups.

- Use a piece of Parmesan rind to impart a dense, savory richness to your soup stock at negligible calorie cost.

And Finally: The Really Lazy Fast Day Diet

If all this cooking sounds like too much of a commitment on a day when you really don't want to think about food, there are options so simple that you barely need to be conscious to get them into your mouth. These include

- Raw vegetables—baby carrots in a bag will do—plus a mini container of hummus

- Low-GI fruit such as strawberries, cherries, apples, and pears (eat the core)

- Unsweetened muesli with skimmed milk

- Weight Watchers Baked Beans

- A cup of bouillon or clear broth

- A hard-boiled egg

- A grab of salad leaves from a bag; thawed shrimp from the freezer; a good squeeze of lemon; salt, pepper, and red pepper flakes

- A pile of lightly steamed vegetables— anything you may find in the fridge—with lots of black pepper and a good grating of Parmesan or pecorino

- A few slices of fat-free ham with a ripe, sliced beefsteak tomato

- Soup from a shop, preferably a light vegetable soup, not a thick cream soup or pasta soup

- Microwavable low-calorie meals. They're an expensive way to get a fast day fix, but the labels are clear and the nutrition should be balanced.

- Other store-bought quickies: if you are nipping out of the office on a fast day, there are good options available, as long as you choose wisely and check the calorie counts.

But, of course, it's so much better to make your own fast day food . . .

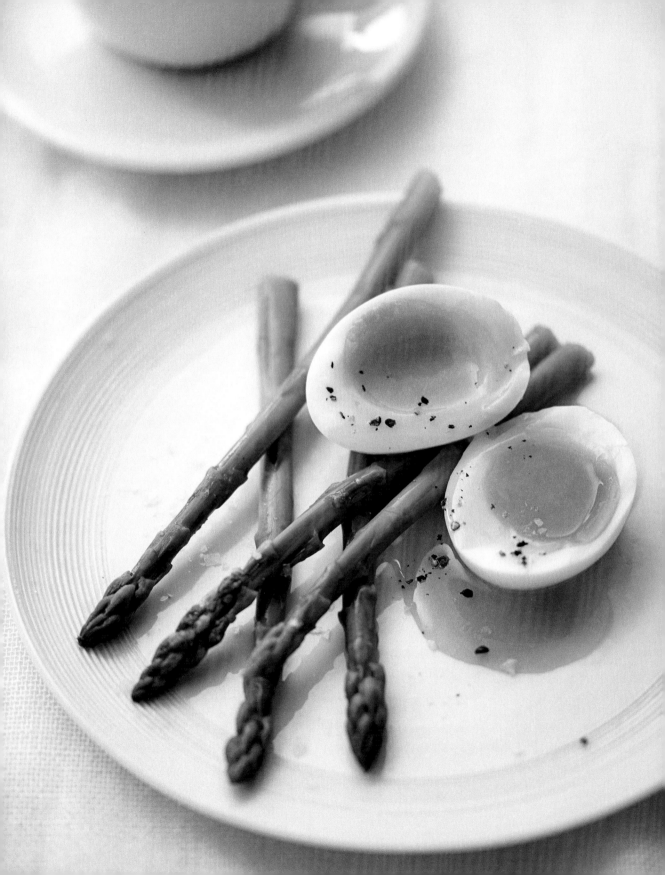

CHAPTER FOUR

simple breakfasts

SOFT-BOILED EGG WITH ASPARAGUS SPEARS

CALORIE COUNT: 90

There's a reason eggs are such a great start to a fast day. They are an incomparable source of good things: healthy fats, protein (all nine essential amino acids), B vitamins, all manner of minerals. Do buy the best you can—free-range chickens have been shown to produce eggs of higher nutritional quality.[1]

Eat them fresh as a daisy, and settle down with asparagus spears in lieu of toast on a spring morning.

Take a medium egg; place in a pan of cold water. Bring to a boil and allow to simmer for 3 to 4 minutes. Take 5 asparagus spears, trim the ends, and either add to the boiling water with the egg, or steam for the 3 to 4 minutes.

NB

ASPARAGUS IS A RICH SOURCE OF FOLATE NEEDED FOR HEALTHY BLOOD.

LEAN EGGS AND HAM

CALORIE COUNT: 118

Poaching or boiling an egg avoids the addition of careless calories. But poaching eggs—like marriage—is a simple business that can quickly get complicated. The method here is the established one, involving a bit of swirling and a dash of vinegar. For a couple of clever alternative methods, and one that allows you to poach eggs in advance, see page 14.

Bring a large pan of lightly salted water to a boil and keep at a simmer over gentle heat. Crack a medium egg into a cup. Swirl the simmering water; add 1½ teaspoons vinegar to help the egg white coagulate; then gently add the egg. Poach for 2 to 3 minutes or till set to your liking. Remove it from the pan with a slotted spoon and set to dry on paper towels. Serve with 2 slices lean ham (⅓ to ½ ounce/10 to 15g each), or with steamed asparagus and a scant grating of Parmesan (about 1 teaspoon).

NB

EGG YOLKS ARE ONE OF THE FEW NATURAL SOURCES OF VITAMIN D IN THE DIET, NECESSARY FOR CALCIUM ABSORPTION AND TO KEEP BONES HEALTHY.

STRAWBERRIES WITH RICOTTA, BLACK PEPPER, AND BALSAMIC

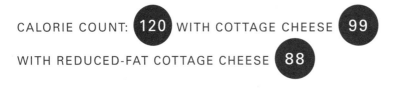

CALORIE COUNT: 120 WITH COTTAGE CHEESE 99

WITH REDUCED-FAT COTTAGE CHEESE 88

Without sugar, strawberries have a low GL and are deliciously low in calories—no wonder many fasters eat a bowlful for breakfast. Adding a spoonful of ricotta cheese gives you light-touch dairy protein, too. Made from whey, ricotta is relatively low in fat, making it a good alternative to mascarpone in other recipes. If you really want to slash your calories, serve your strawberries with a small mound of cottage cheese.

15 fresh strawberries
Scant 2 ounces/50g full-fat ricotta
A grind of black pepper
A dash of balsamic vinegar, or to taste

Assemble prettily on a plate and dig in.

NB

STRAWBERRIES CONTAIN ANTIOXIDANTS CALLED ANTHOCYANINS, WHICH MAY HAVE ANTICARCINOGENIC PROPERTIES[2] . . . THEY ALSO HAVE A VERY LOW GL OF 3.

SMOKED SALMON WITH CAPERS AND RED ONION

CALORIE COUNT: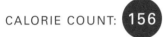

A classic, of course, best served with plenty of lemon. Smoked salmon provides plenty of protein, together with important omega-3 fatty acids that can help keep the heart healthy. The capers and red onion here will help cut through the smooth oiliness of the fish. For me, the whole event feels like a bit of a treat, which is no bad thing on a fast day.

3½ ounces/100g smoked salmon
1 teaspoon drained capers
¼ small red onion, thinly sliced
Juice of ½ lemon

Place the salmon on a plate and garnish with the capers, sliced onion, and lemon juice.

NB

SALMON PROVIDES SELENIUM, A TRACE MINERAL THAT HELPS TO PROTECT AGAINST FREE RADICAL DAMAGE.

WATERMELON, FRESH FIG, AND PROSCIUTTO

CALORIE COUNT: 185

Although melons and watermelons tend to be high in sugar, they have a low GL. Watermelon scores a GL of 4, which matches that of apples. Figs are full of fiber (if you eat the skin and seeds), and they're uncommonly pretty, too: a pretty plate is, generally speaking, a healthy one. A couple of slices of prosciutto make this a classic combination, and will deliver a jolt of protein to kick-start the day.

Take a large slice of watermelon (about 7 ounces/200g), seed, dice, and serve with a fresh fig and 2 slices of prosciutto.

NB

FIGS CONTAIN USEFUL MINERALS SUCH AS CALCIUM AND MAGNESIUM.

SLICED APPLE WITH CINNAMON DIP

CALORIE COUNT: 223

Apples are the ultimate convenience food, though they are quite high in calories. Eat the whole thing—skin, seeds, and core—to get maximum fiber.

1 apple, thinly sliced, with a squeeze of lemon
½ cup/100g crème fraîche or fromage blanc
½ teaspoon honey
A sprinkling of ground cinnamon

Assemble in a bowl and dig in.

NB

PECTIN IN APPLES LIMITS THE AMOUNT OF FAT THAT CELLS CAN ABSORB, HELPS BALANCE BLOOD SUGAR LEVELS, AND CAUSES THE STOMACH TO EMPTY MORE SLOWLY, LEAVING YOU FULLER LONGER.[3]

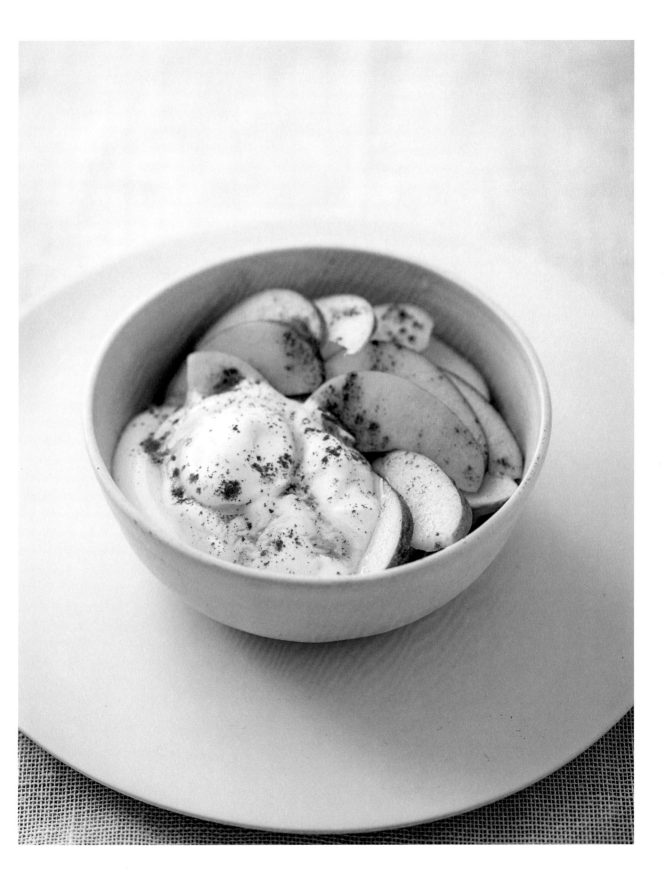

YOGURT WITH PLUM, BLANCHED ALMONDS, AND AGAVE NECTAR

CALORIE COUNT: 264

Yogurt has long been considered a "health food"—and it is packed with calcium, B vitamins, and friendly bacteria. On a fast day, choose wisely: Fruit yogurts can be high in fat and hidden sugars, so go for a low-fat unflavored version and boost the taste with fresh plums. They are relatively low-calorie and a good source of fiber, which makes them brilliantly satiating.

½ cup/100g unflavored low-fat yogurt
2 plums, pitted and sliced
1 level tablespoon/20g blanched almonds
2 teaspoons raw agave nectar

The ingredients look gorgeous when layered in a glass tumbler. The only other thing you need is a spoon.

NB

ALMONDS ARE A RICH SOURCE OF MAGNESIUM (YOU'LL GET A THIRD OF YOUR RDA FROM JUST 10 OF THEM)—GREAT FOR THE NERVOUS SYSTEM.

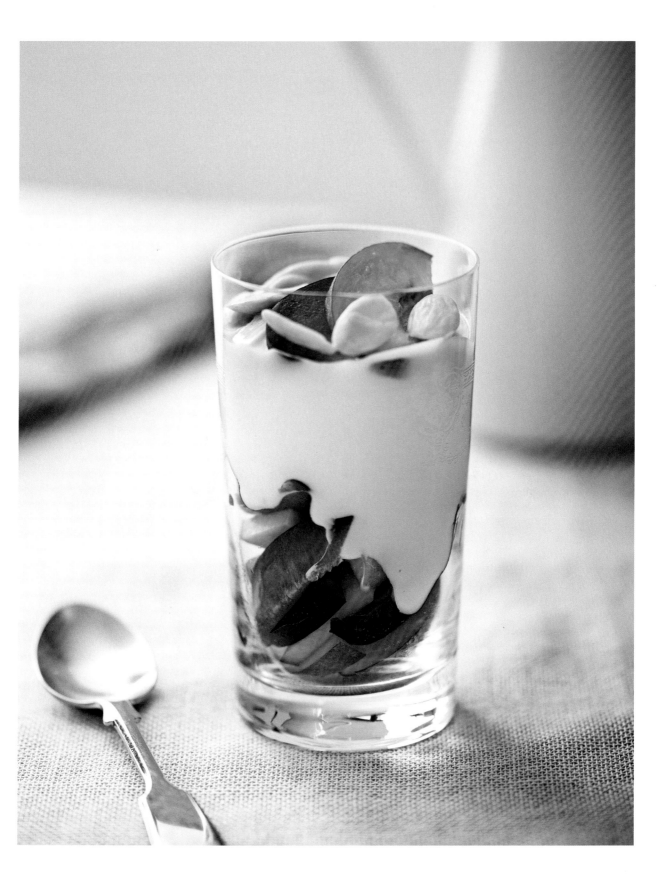

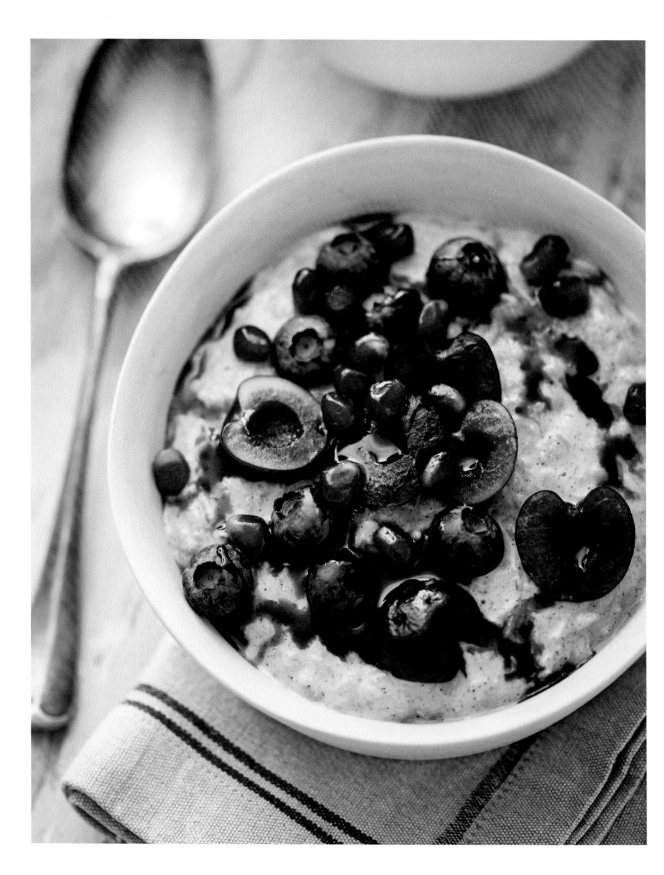

OATMEAL WITH JEWEL FRUITS

CALORIE COUNT: 284

Add a delicate swirl of pomegranate molasses, along with pomegranate seeds and a dusting of cinnamon, to arrive at a wonderful, ruby-studded dish with a flash of inspiration from the Middle East. Use old-fashioned oatmeal as it will keep you fuller longer than the more processed varieties.

1¼ cups/300ml skimmed milk
1 ounce/30g old-fashioned oatmeal
½ teaspoon ground cinnamon
A pinch of salt
1 teaspoon pomegranate molasses
Scant 2 ounces/50g fruit of choice (stick to the lower-GI fruits such as berries and cherries)

Heat the milk, oats, cinnamon, and salt in a small saucepan. Stir well till the oatmeal is thickened, 4 to 5 minutes (you can do this in a microwave, stirring halfway through the 5-minute cooking time). Leave to stand for a minute before adding the molasses and fruit.

NB

THE FIBER IN OATS CAN HELP TO LOWER BLOOD CHOLESTEROL.

SCRAMBLED EGGS WITH SMOKED SALMON

CALORIE COUNT: 303

There are some things that cry out for butter. Scrambled eggs are, in my opinion, one of them, so use it here, but sparingly. The pairing with smoked salmon is, of course, a classic and doesn't really need to be fiddled with. The furthest I'd go is adding a scatter of chives.

2 medium eggs
Salt and pepper
Minced chives
½ teaspoon/5g butter
3 ounces/80g smoked salmon, slivered

Beat the eggs with the salt and pepper. Whisking well, add the chives. Melt the butter in a small nonstick pan and cook the eggs very gently, stirring all the time. Remove from heat and serve immediately with slivers of salmon.

NB

THIS BREAKFAST DELIVERS OVER 30G OF PROTEIN, WHICH SHOULD HELP YOU FEEL FULLER FOR LONGER.

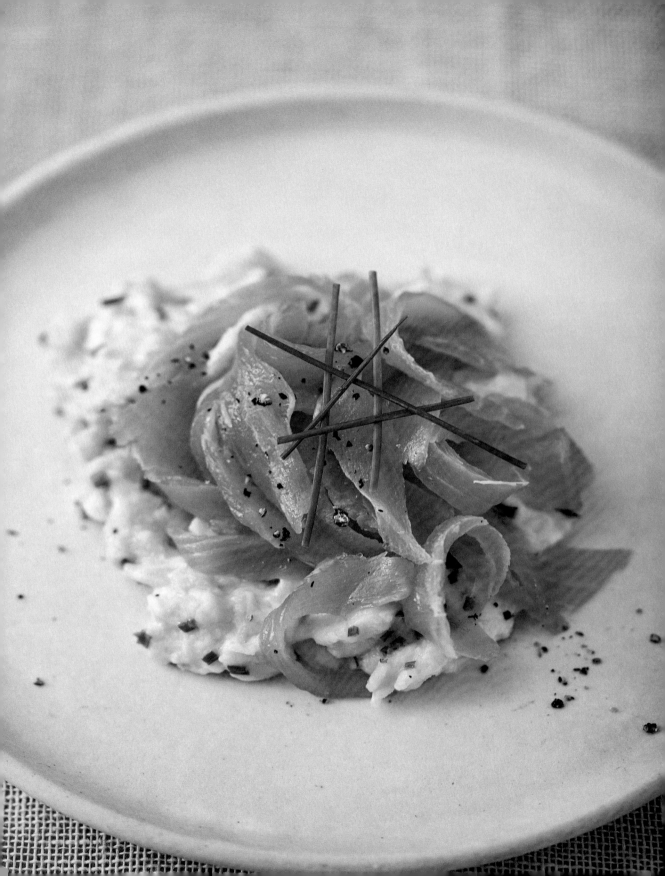

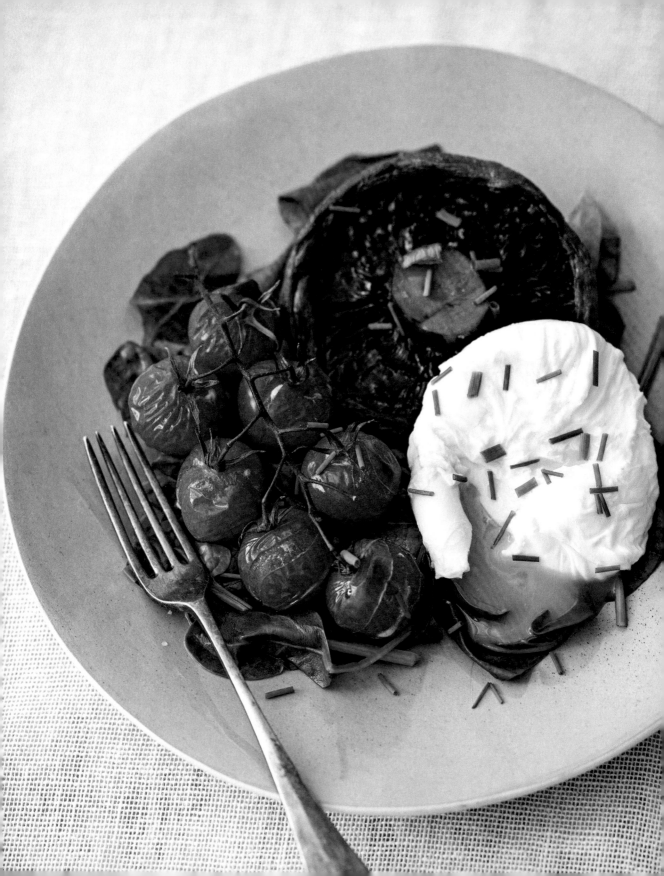

CHAPTER FIVE

leisurely breakfasts

POACHED EGGS WITH SPINACH, PORTOBELLO MUSHROOM, AND CHERRY TOMATOES

CALORIE COUNT: 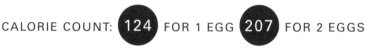 **124** FOR 1 EGG **207** FOR 2 EGGS

Research recently found that people who consume egg protein for breakfast are more likely to feel full during the day than those whose breakfasts contain wheat protein,[1] so an omelet makes fast day sense. It's the combination of plants and proteins that makes this dish such a successful fast day breakfast. That, and the delicious taste—all for obligingly few calories.

Salt and pepper
1 large portobello mushroom cap
6 to 8 cherry tomatoes (preferably on the vine)
Spray oil
1 or 2 medium eggs
3½ ounces/100g baby spinach leaves
A pinch of nutmeg
Minced chives

Season the mushroom and tomatoes, spray with a little oil, and place under a hot broiler for 5 minutes. Poach the eggs for 3 to 4 minutes (page 14). Meanwhile, wilt the spinach in a saucepan, drain, and add a pinch of nutmeg. Serve garnished with chives.

NB

SPINACH IS PACKED WITH VITAMINS AND MINERALS, INCLUDING FOLATE AND IRON.

SHAKSHOUKA

CALORIE COUNT: 178

This is a delicious feast, originally Tunisian, of eggs poached in a cumin-infused tomato concassé. Studies have shown that lycopene, a red pigment and potent antioxidant found in tomatoes, is boosted in cooking,[2] so you are maximizing your nutritional benefit with this slow-cooked sauce. The recipe here is for two, as it tends to work better when cooked in a larger pan. Simply halve the quantities and use a small, heavy pan if you're cooking for one.

Serves 2

1½ teaspoons olive oil
½ medium onion, peeled and diced
1 clove garlic, minced
1 medium red bell pepper, chopped
One 14-ounce/400g can diced tomatoes
1 tablespoon tomato paste
½ teaspoon paprika
½ teaspoon mild chili powder
½ teaspoon ground cumin
A pinch of cayenne pepper
Salt and pepper
2 medium eggs
1½ teaspoons chopped fresh parsley

Heat a medium sauté pan and warm the olive oil. Add the onion and sauté for a few minutes till the onion begins to soften. Add the garlic and bell pepper and cook for 5 to 7 minutes over medium heat till softened. Stir in the tomatoes and tomato paste, together with the spices, and simmer for 5 to 7 minutes more, till it starts to reduce. Season with salt and pepper, then crack the eggs directly over the tomato mixture. Cover and cook for 10 minutes, till the egg whites are firm, the yolks are still runny, and the sauce has slightly reduced. Garnish with flurries of chopped parsley.

NB

THIS BREAKFAST PROVIDES DOUBLE THE RDA OF VITAMIN C.

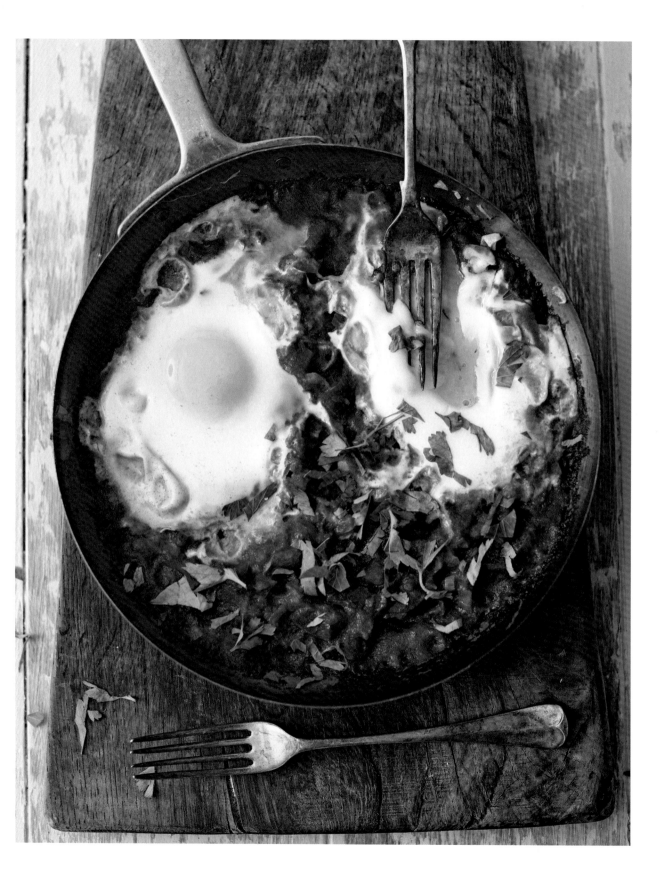

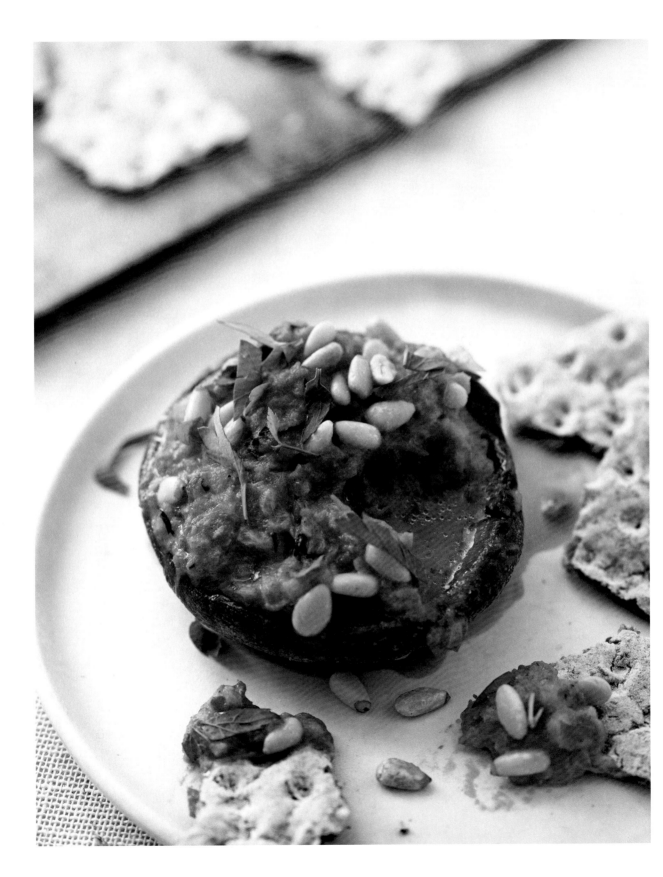

MUSHROOM, PEPPER, AND TOMATO CONCASSÉ WITH THIN RYE CRISPBREAD

CALORIE COUNT: 181

This is another showstopper, a real "come-over-to-my-place" breakfast or brunch, which means you can follow your fast without anyone else knowing about it. Make plenty of the concassé—you can double or even triple the recipe—and use it another way on another day. It will keep in the fridge for 3 to 4 days and it freezes well. The concassé recipe here makes enough for four servings.

Tomato concassé
2 red bell peppers
1 tablespoon olive oil
2 cloves garlic, minced
1 shallot, diced
4 large, ripe tomatoes, diced
2 tablespoons fresh basil leaves
1 teaspoon fresh oregano leaves
Salt and pepper
2 tablespoons water

Mushroom base and garnish
1 medium portobello mushroom cap
1 teaspoon pine nuts, toasted
Salt and pepper
Fresh flat-leaf parsley, chopped
2 thin rye crispbreads, such as Wasa

Start with the concassé. Roast the bell peppers in a hot oven (400°F) until browned. Leave the oven on. Chop, seed, and set aside. Heat the olive oil in a small saucepan, add the garlic and shallot, and sweat till softened. Add the tomatoes, herbs, roasted peppers, salt and pepper, and water and cook for 8 to 10 minutes, till gently reduced. Allow to cool slightly, then blend in a food processor or with a stick blender till coarsely combined.

Bake mushroom in a baking pan for 3 to 5 minutes. Spoon concassé into the central well of the mushroom. Bake for an additional 5 minutes. Sprinkle with toasted pine nuts, season with salt and pepper, and serve with chopped parsley and crispbread dippers.

NB

MUSHROOMS ARE A GOOD SOURCE OF B VITAMINS, PLUS THE VITAL MINERALS SELENIUM, COPPER, AND POTASSIUM.

FLUFFED SHRIMP OMELET

CALORIE COUNT:

The fluffing here won't do anything to reduce the calorie count—the world doesn't work like that—but it does look great and it certainly assists, together with the bulk of the zucchini and protein from the shrimp, in making a substantial breakfast. This a good one to serve to nonfasting friends on your fast day. Let them have hot buttered toast with theirs, knowing that you can have yours tomorrow.

1 ounce/30g cooked and peeled shrimp
½ zucchini, grated and wrung dry
2 medium eggs, separated
A dash of Tabasco sauce
Salt and pepper
Spray oil
Flat-leaf parsley sprig to serve

Dry the shrimp on paper towels and mix with the grated zucchini. Whisk the egg whites till stiff peaks form. Beat the egg yolks with the Tabasco, salt, and pepper. With a metal spoon, gently fold the egg yolk mixture into the whisked whites. Heat a pan and spray with a little oil. Fry the shrimp mixture for a minute or two, then add the eggs and cook till the omelet is set. Finish under the broiler if you prefer a firmer texture. Serve with torn parsley.

NB

EGG YOLKS ARE ONE OF THE FEW NATURAL SOURCES OF VITAMIN D IN THE DIET, NECESSARY FOR CALCIUM ABSORPTION AND TO KEEP BONES HEALTHY.

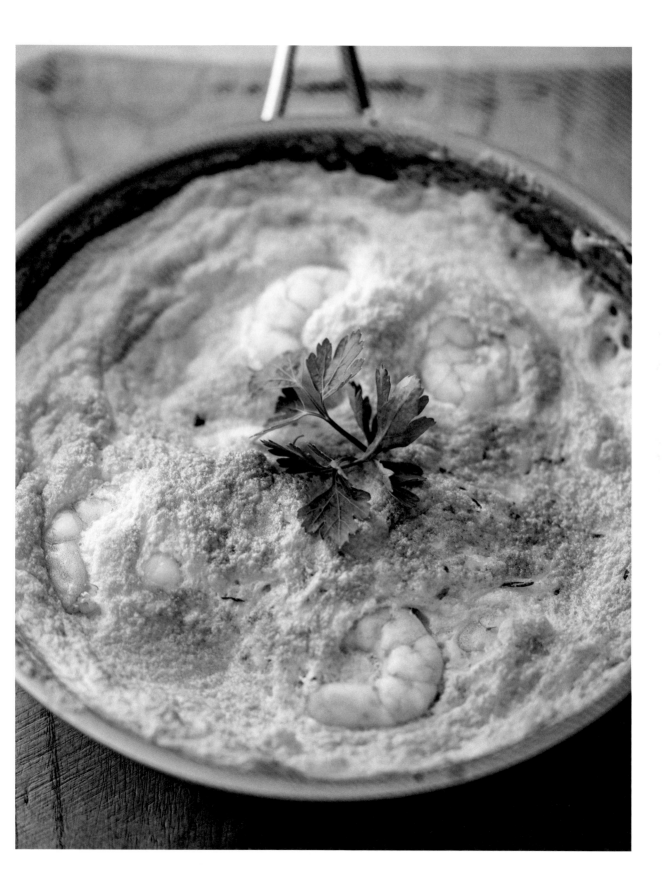

FAST DAY MUESLI WITH FRESH CHERRY OR STRAWBERRY YOGURT

CALORIE COUNT: 223

Store-bought mueslis not only tend to contain sugary dried fruit, they generally include something you don't like very much and have to pick out before you get a dream mouthful. So make your own low-GI muesli with plenty of seeds and nuts and coconut for sweetness. Stick with it: Once you've trained your taste buds to enjoy this infinitely superior fast day version, the sugared varieties will start to taste oversweet.

Muesli
3½ ounces/100g whole oat flakes
1 ounce/30g oat bran
2 tablespoons sunflower seeds
2 tablespoons pumpkin seeds
2 tablespoons flaxseed
2 tablespoons poppy seeds
2 tablespoons almonds
2 tablespoons hazelnuts
2 tablespoons unsweetened dried coconut flakes
Scant 2 ounces/50g ground almonds

Base and topping
½ cup/100g unflavored low-fat yogurt
10 ripe cherries, pitted, or 10 ripe strawberries, husked

Mix the muesli ingredients and keep in an airtight container. (You can, of course, multiply the quantities.) Place the low-fat yogurt in a bowl and add a handful of the muesli, then top with fruit.

NB

COCONUT IS RICH IN POTASSIUM, WHICH CAN HELP KEEP BLOOD PRESSURE HEALTHY.

HIGH-ENERGY BREAKFAST

CALORIE COUNT: 246

Cameron Diaz apparently eats her supper at breakfast time—this, she says, keeps her going all day: "I started doing it when I'd go surfing because I could go out for four hours and not get hungry." So if you're a big breakfast person, try an upside-down day— if you can face frying garlic in the morning.

Serves 2

1½ teaspoons olive oil
2 skinless, boneless chicken breasts, cut into ¾-inch cubes
Salt and pepper
3½ ounces/100g broccoli, thinly sliced
3½ ounces/100g cooked brown rice (cook the rice in stock for better flavor)
2 cloves garlic, chopped
1 tablespoon grated lemon zest
1 whole medium egg plus 1 medium egg white, scrambled
2 tablespoons fresh lemon juice
A handful of fresh parsley, chopped

Heat a large skillet and put in the olive oil. Add the chicken and season. Cook for 3 minutes, stirring occasionally. Add the broccoli and continue cooking for 5 minutes more or till the chicken begins to brown. Add cooked rice, garlic, and lemon zest; cook for 3 minutes more. Scramble the egg and egg white in a separate pan and add to the mixture. Heat for 2 minutes more till the chicken is cooked through. Remove from the heat and add lemon juice and plenty of parsley.

NB

THE CALCIUM IN BROCCOLI IS MORE READILY ABSORBED THAN THAT IN OTHER GREEN VEGGIES.

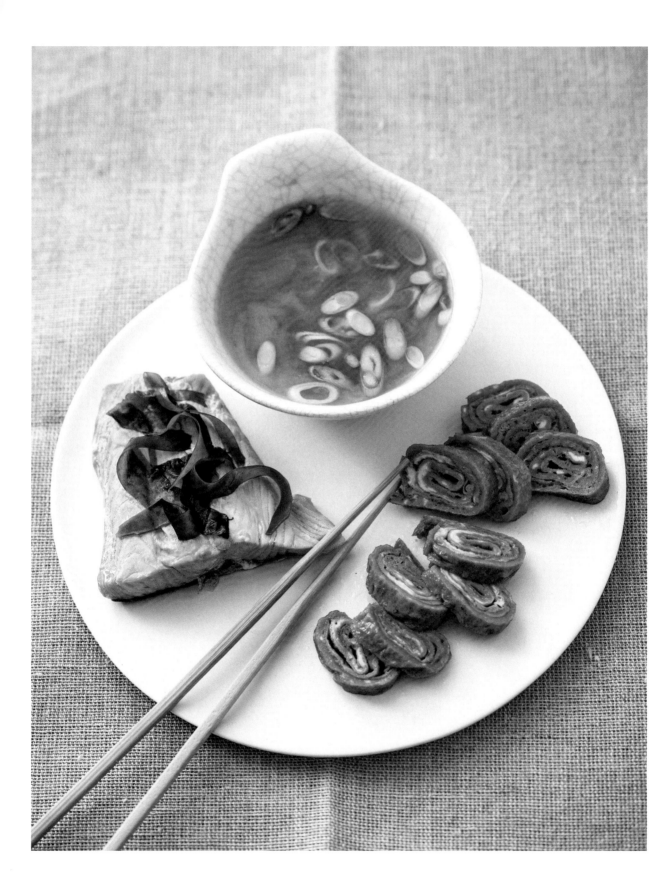

JAPANESE BREAKFAST SPECIAL

CALORIE COUNT FOR THE WHOLE BREAKFAST PER PERSON: 261

This is a fast day take on a traditional Japanese breakfast, boycotting the rice but sticking to the basic components of miso soup, rolled omelet, and steamed fish. It's quite hands-on, so one for a lazy morning. Traditional accompaniments include *tsukemono* (pickles) such as *umeboshi* plums, *natto* (fermented soybeans), nori (dried seaweed strips), and shredded cabbage. Serve with green tea.

Serves 2

Miso Soup

CALORIE COUNT: 78

According to legend, miso was a gift from the gods to ensure humanity's health, longevity, and happiness. I have no reason to argue. This works as a quick and healthy snack, too, if your fast is faltering.

1¼ cups/300ml dashi soup stock (page 178)
2 tablespoons miso paste
3½ ounces/100g tofu, cut into chunks
1 scallion (green onion), thinly sliced on the diagonal

Mix 1 tablespoon dashi stock with miso paste till it dissolves; set aside. Heat the rest of the dashi till boiling, lower the heat to a simmer, and add the tofu. Let cook for 10 minutes. Add the miso mixture and stir. Remove from the heat before it starts boiling. Add the scallion and serve.

Tamagoyaki (Rolled Omelet)

CALORIE COUNT: 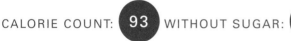 93 WITHOUT SUGAR: 77

The traditional rolled omelet is slightly sweet, which may be an acquired taste. Exclude the sugar to arrive at a Western version (your calorie count will be reduced by about 16 calories).

2 medium eggs
1 teaspoon sugar
1½ teaspoons mirin
1½ teaspoons soy sauce
Salt and pepper
3 tablespoons dashi
Vegetable oil

Break the eggs into a small bowl. Beat with a fork, then add the sugar, mirin, soy sauce, salt and pepper, and dashi. Blend well. Heat the pan with a little oil and pour in half the egg mixture. When it starts to set, roll it and shift to one side of the pan. Repeat with the rest of the egg mixture in the remaining part of the pan and let it spread under the first roll. As it starts to set, roll it over the first one. Once it is fully cooked, remove the omelet from the pan and cut into bite-size pieces.

Steamed Salmon

CALORIE COUNT: 90

3½ ounces/100g fresh salmon

Steam the fish lightly till cooked to your liking.

NB

THIS BREAKFAST IS FULL OF MINERAL MAGIC—AND A SOUP FOR BREAKFAST HAS BEEN PROVED TO KEEP YOU FULLER LONGER.[3]

BEAUTY BREAKFAST SHAKE

CALORIE COUNT: 279

This makes a cool and pleasantly DIY shake, full of goodies—a bit of a belly boost to start the day. Because you're in charge here, there's no danger of consuming the hidden sugars and preservatives that tend to lurk in many commercial products.

½ cup unflavored low-fat yogurt

1 ounce/30g old-fashioned oatmeal

1 teaspoon sunflower seeds

1½ tablespoons/20g chopped dried apricots

1½ ounces/20g blanched almonds, chopped

Mix the yogurt with water till the consistency of a shake. Combine with the remaining ingredients in a bowl or large glass and leave in the fridge overnight, ready for a breakfast boost.

NB

SEEDS AND NUTS ARE A SOURCE OF HEALTHY PLANT FATS, AND A GREAT WAY TO START THE DAY.

SPICED PEAR PORRIDGE

CALORIE COUNT: 221 WITH AGAVE 299

The spice and fruit here help make up for the lack of added sugar. Oats are full of soluble fiber and release energy slowly to set you up for the day. Add the chopped hazelnuts and agave nectar (a low-GI sweetener, now widely available) as a topping if your calorie count allows.

1 ounce/30g old-fashioned oatmeal

1 cup/250ml skimmed milk

½ pear, peeled and sliced

½ teaspoon ground cinnamon

A grating of nutmeg

1 tablespoon chopped hazelnuts

1 teaspoon agave nectar

Place the oats, milk, pear, cinnamon, and nutmeg in a saucepan and simmer, stirring, till the oatmeal is thickened to your liking. Serve with the nuts, adding a little agave nectar to taste.

NB

OATS ARE SLOW-BURNING AND SPACE-FILLING; THEY ARE HEART-HEALTHY AND ANTIOXIDANT, TOO.[4]

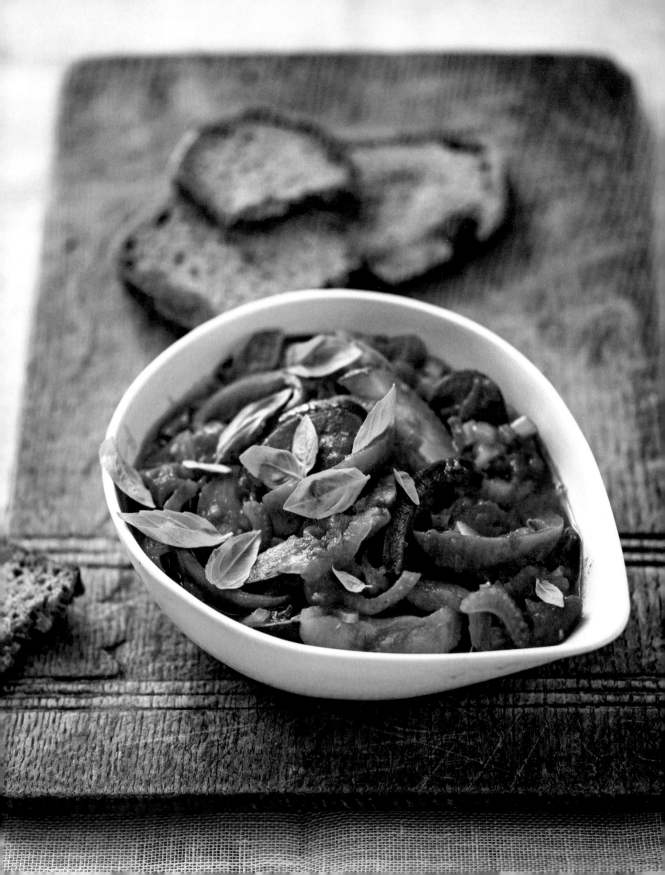

simple suppers

RATATOUILLE WITH RYE TOAST

CALORIE COUNT: **118** WITH RYE TOAST **173**

Most of us know how to make ratatouille, chiefly because it's one of those cheerful dishes that can cope with anything you sling at it. I've slung plenty at this version, in order to max out the veggie content. Don't leave out the tiny amount of sugar here—it helps to bring out the flavor in any cooked tomato dish. Make this in double quantity and have it handy in the freezer for a fast day fix.

Serves 4

2 onions, sliced
1½ teaspoons olive oil
2 cloves garlic, minced
1 stalk celery, finely chopped
2 green bell peppers, sliced into strips
2 small eggplants, sliced
2 zucchini, cut into chunks
Two 14-ounce/400g cans diced tomatoes
1 teaspoon dried oregano
½ teaspoon red pepper flakes
½ teaspoon sugar
Salt and pepper
Scant ½ cup/100ml water
A handful of fresh basil leaves, for garnish
4 thin slices rye bread, toasted

Sauté the onion in the oil till softened and translucent. Add the garlic and celery and cook for 2 minutes more. Add the bell peppers and cook for 3 minutes. Add the eggplants, zucchini, tomatoes, oregano, red pepper, sugar, salt and pepper, and water, and cook for 30 minutes, stirring occasionally, adding more water if necessary to achieve the correct consistency. Serve at room temperature, topped with basil leaves and with a thin slice of crisply toasted rye bread.

NB

ONE PORTION OF RATATOUILLE WILL PROVIDE THREE OF YOUR FIVE-A-DAY VEGETABLE SERVINGS.

BEEF CARPACCIO WITH LEMON-DRESSED HERBS

CALORIE COUNT: WITH 1 TEASPOON OLIVE OIL

If you are feeling adventurous, try this (typically at less calorie cost) with venison. Whatever you choose, use only the freshest, finest, leanest meat. You're not eating much of it, so make it matter.

3½ ounces/100g beef filet
A squeeze of lemon juice
3 ounces/80g baby arugula leaves
Salt and cracked black pepper
A drizzle of olive oil (optional)

Sear the beef for the briefest time in a very hot pan. Chill, then slice paper-thin. Lay the delicate slices of beef on a plate. Dress with lemon juice, arugula leaves, flakes of salt, and a generous grind of black pepper. A drizzle of good-quality olive oil would make things perfect.

NB

LEAN BEEF IS A GOOD SOURCE OF EASILY ABSORBED IRON, VITAL FOR HEALTHY BLOOD.

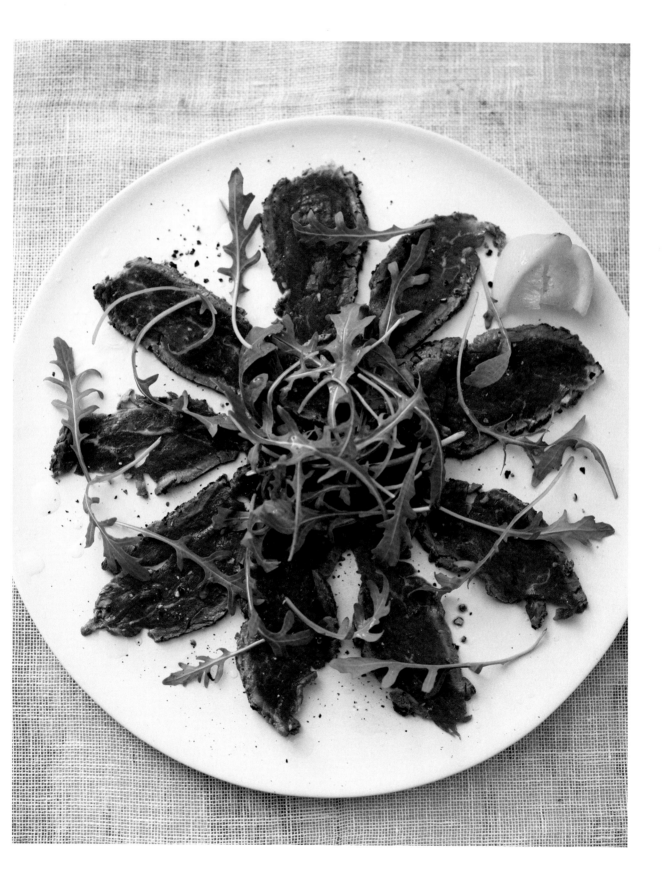

STANDBY VEGGIE CHILI

CALORIE COUNT: **149** WITH A TACO SHELL: **199**

A standard way to ferry vegetables into your mouth in a vehicle of fabulous full-on flavor. Don't be too prescriptive here—this is not a bean-counting exercise. And do have the taco shell; a bit of crunch on a fast day can be welcome indeed. This is another freezer-friendly dish.

Serves 4

1 onion, diced
1 teaspoon olive oil
2 cloves garlic, minced
2 red chiles, seeded and finely chopped
2 teaspoons ground cumin
Salt and pepper
Scant pinch of sugar
5 ounces/150g mushrooms, chopped
One 14-ounce/400g can diced tomatoes
One 14-ounce/400g can red kidney beans, drained
1 tablespoon tomato paste
3½ ounces/100g green beans, blanched and chopped
A handful of fresh cilantro, chopped
4 corn taco shells

Sauté the onion in the olive oil for a few minutes till softened. Add the garlic, chiles, cumin, salt, pepper, and sugar. Add the mushrooms, tomatoes, kidney beans, and tomato paste, stir, and simmer for 10 minutes. Add the green beans and cook to heat through. Serve with a scatter of cilantro in a corn taco shell (which has a low GL of 8 and about 50 calories).

NB

LEAVE MUSHROOMS ON A WINDOWSILL TO EXPOSE THEM TO SUNLIGHT; THIS WILL BOOST THEIR VITAMIN D CONTENT.

For a chili con Quorn, use crumbled Quorn instead of, or in addition to, the mushrooms.

WARM PUY LENTILS WITH TOMATOES AND CRUMBLED FETA

CALORIE COUNT: **153**

This is one of my all-time favorite recipes and standard fare in our house. Generally I make it as a side dish for barbecues, but it works equally well as a main dish, particularly on a fast day. Lentils have been part of the human diet since Neolithic times, and with good reason: They are high in protein, fiber, vitamin B, and other vitals such as iron and folate—and because they release their energy slowly, they help to keep blood sugar levels in check.

Serves 4

3½ ounces/100g Puy lentils, rinsed (or use brown or
    green lentils)
½ teaspoon red wine vinegar
1 clove garlic, peeled and left whole, plus ½ clove, finely chopped
1 bay leaf
3 peppercorns
A pinch of sugar
2 cups/475ml cold water
1 medium red onion, finely chopped
2 ripe tomatoes, chopped
1 tablespoon balsamic vinegar
1 tablespoon olive oil
Scant 2 ounces/50g feta cheese, crumbled
Salt and pepper
A large handful of flat-leaf parsley, chopped

Place the lentils in a pan with the vinegar, whole garlic clove, bay leaf, peppercorns, and sugar. Cover with cold water. Bring to a boil and simmer for 20 minutes or till lentils are tender but retain their shape. Drain, discard the garlic, bay leaf, and peppercorns, and leave to cool slightly. Mix the remaining ingredients and stir through the warm lentils. Season well and serve with plenty of parsley.

NB

THE VITAMIN C FROM THE PARSLEY AND TOMATOES WILL HELP THE ABSORPTION OF THE IRON IN THE LENTILS.

YOUNG YELLOW SQUASH WITH FETA, LEMON ZEST, AND MINT

CALORIE COUNT: 156

It's the combination of ingredients here that really makes for something special, the kind of thing you might eat on the terrace of a restaurant overlooking the Aegean . . .

Make sure the squash is grilled well and properly marked—that's all part of the presentation.

1 teaspoon olive oil
2 yellow squash, sliced lengthwise into strips
Salt and pepper
A handful of young fresh mint leaves
1½ ounces/40g feta cheese, crumbled
Zest of 1 lemon
A squeeze of lemon juice
Baby arugula leaves, for serving

Heat a cast-iron grill pan. Brush oil on the squash strips, season, and grill, turning once, till they are prettily striped, 3 to 4 minutes per side. Don't overcrowd the pan. Serve topped with mint, feta, lemon zest curls, and a squeeze of lemon, with an arugula salad on the side.

NB

ALL SUMMER SQUASH IS A GOOD SOURCE OF VITAMIN A, BUT THE YELLOW ONES CONTAIN MORE OF THE VITAMIN THAN MOST.

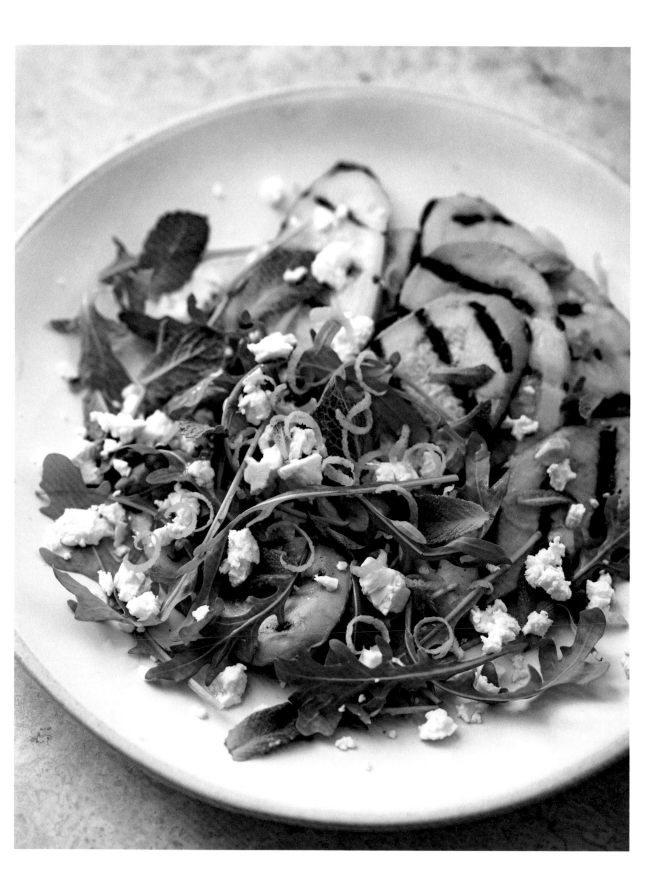

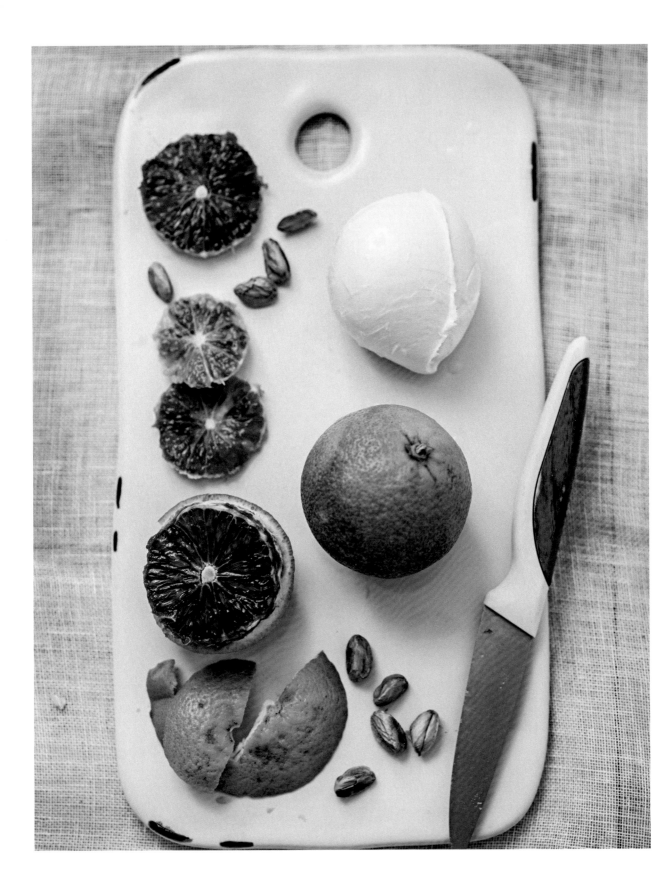

FAST DAY TRICOLORE THREE WAYS

Who can argue with a tricolore? It may well be the most visually gratifying triumvirate of ingredients ever gathered together on a plate. It does matter for taste, however, that your tomatoes are good ones and that your mozzarella is milky and sensitive to the touch. Part-skim mozzarella will probably have to do for a fast day, but this is a small price to pay for eating such incomparable deliciousness.

Classic

CALORIE COUNT: 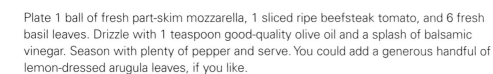 **158**

Plate 1 ball of fresh part-skim mozzarella, 1 sliced ripe beefsteak tomato, and 6 fresh basil leaves. Drizzle with 1 teaspoon good-quality olive oil and a splash of balsamic vinegar. Season with plenty of pepper and serve. You could add a generous handful of lemon-dressed arugula leaves, if you like.

Roasted

CALORIE COUNT: **144**

Roast 6 to 8 cherry tomatoes, preferably on the vine, in a hot oven for 10 minutes or till the skins just burst. Serve with basil leaves and part-skim mozzarella, and drizzle with a tablespoon of black olive tapenade, thinned with 1 teaspoon olive oil.

Blood Orange, Arugula, and Pistachios

CALORIE COUNT: **180**

For a grand and glorious alternative, try tricolore with reduced-fat buffalo mozzarella, blood orange segments, wisps of arugula, and 10 to 12 shelled pistachios, all seasoned with salt and pepper and dressed with 1 teaspoon blood orange juice and 1 teaspoon olive oil.

NB

PISTACHIOS CONTAIN MORE POTASSIUM THAN ANY OTHER NUT.

SASHIMI WITH WASABI AND PICKLED GINGER

CALORIE COUNT: 196

It stands to reason that the pure protein of sashimi is a fast day friend, if you pick your fish with care and consideration. Make sure that it is super fresh—clear-eyed, silver scaled—and slice it with a very sharp knife. That way, it is a thing of beauty and a joy for about 3 minutes—it won't last long before your chopsticks get to work.

3½ ounces/100g raw tuna, halibut, or salmon, very fresh and sliced very thin
Wasabi paste, soy sauce, and pickled ginger, for serving

Place the fish slices on a plate. Garnish with wasabi, soy sauce, and ginger, or serve them on the side.

NB

SASHIMI IS A GOOD SOURCE OF IODINE, A REGULATOR OF METABOLIC RATE.

As a great fast day alternative, try Italian *crudo*. Take 3½ ounces/100g super fresh raw ocean fish (such as line-caught bass, bream, or mackerel) and slice it paper thin. (A sharp Japanese knife, with its slimmer 15-degree angled blade, is useful here.) Serve with a drizzle of olive oil, lemon, and fresh herbs rather than the Japanese accompaniments.

TORTILLA PIZZETTA THREE WAYS

Okay, I'm not about to convince you that this equates to a deep-dish pizza with all the trimmings and extra cheese. But it is a light and pleasing way to entertain your taste buds come 7:00 p.m. on a fast day. Make up your own toppings as you go along, avoiding the obvious heavyweights like pepperoni. If you want it Hawaiian, be our guest.

Base

1 whole-grain tortilla
2 tablespoons tomato puree
Salt and pepper

Top the tortilla with the tomato puree and season with salt and pepper. Add one of the toppings and broil for 3 to 4 minutes (or about 5 minutes to melt the cheese).

Tapenade, Pine Nut, and Marjoram

CALORIE COUNT: 196

1 tablespoon store-bought tapenade
1 teaspoon toasted pine nuts
Fresh or dried marjoram

NB

PINE NUTS ARE ONE OF THE RICHEST NATURAL SOURCES OF VITAMIN E, WHILE OLIVES CONTAIN HEALTHY MONOUNSATURATED FATS, GOOD FOR THE HEART.

Mozzarella and Pesto

CALORIE COUNT: 203

½ ball part-skim mozzarella
2 teaspoons pesto, store-bought or homemade
   (page 210)
Torn basil leaves
A drizzle of olive oil

NB

YOU STILL GET PLENTY OF CALCIUM FROM LOW-FAT CHEESE.

Feta and Black Olive

CALORIE COUNT: 218

3 tablespoons crumbled feta cheese
6 black olives, chopped
Fresh oregano and mint leaves

NB

OLIVES CONTAIN HEALTHY MONOUNSATURATED FATS, GOOD FOR THE HEART.

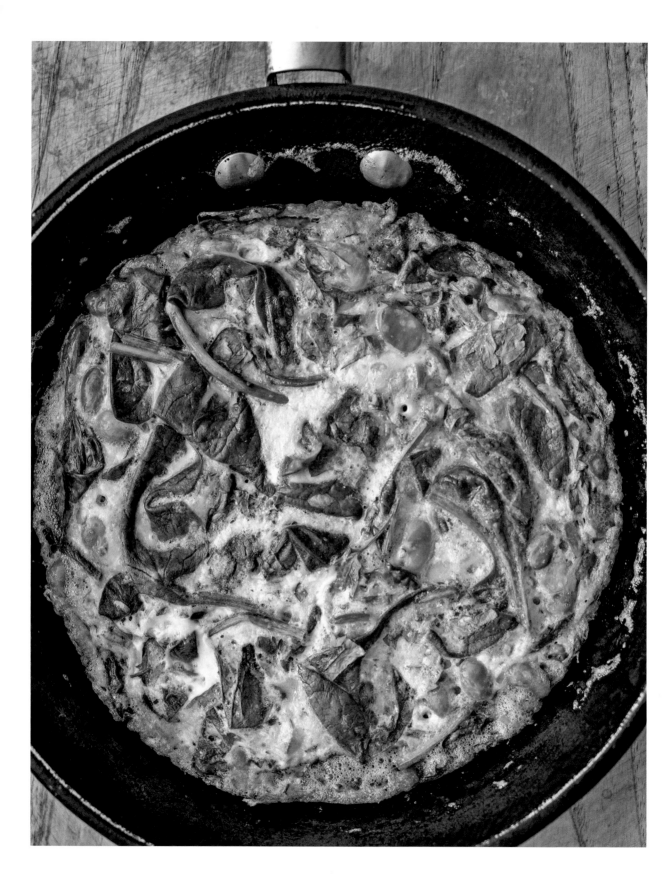

TWO-EGG OMELET FOUR WAYS

An omelet makes a power-packed supper, especially if you combine it with the greens and proteins that lend your fast day a bit of stamina. The 2-egg recipes will work equally well as a substantial breakfast. If you want to cut back on calories, a 1-egg omelet is still a very fine thing. Or a 1-yolk, 2-white omelet can give you a bit more substance without the calories.

Fresh Pea, Smoked Trout, and Dill

CALORIE COUNT: **219**

2 medium eggs
Scant 1 ounce/25g blanched shelled fresh peas
1 ounce/30g smoked trout, flaked
1 teaspoon minced fresh dill
Pepper
Spray oil

Beat the eggs. Stir in the peas, trout, and dill and season with pepper.
Spray your pan and heat over low heat. Pour in the eggs and cook till just set.

Zucchini, Goat Cheese, and Red Onion

CALORIE COUNT: **284**

2 medium eggs
1 small zucchini, grated (squeeze out excess water)
1 ounce/30g minced red onion
Salt and pepper
Spray oil
1 ounce/30g soft goat cheese

Beat the eggs. Stir in the zucchini and onion and season with salt and pepper. Spray your pan and heat over low heat. Pour in the eggs and cook till just set. Top with the cheese and broil for 3 to 4 minutes to melt.

Wilted Spinach, Fava Beans, and Pecorino

CALORIE COUNT: 297

2 medium eggs
3½ ounces/100g shelled fresh or frozen fava beans, blanched
2¼ ounces/60g baby spinach leaves, blanched (see note)
Chopped fresh flat-leaf parsley
1 tablespoon grated pecorino cheese
Salt and pepper
Spray oil

Beat the eggs. Stir in the beans, spinach, parsley, and cheese. Season with salt and pepper. Spray your pan and cook the eggs over low heat till just set. This can be eaten hot or cold, and it's very good for picnics and lunch boxes.

Swiss, Tomato, and Arugula

CALORIE COUNT: 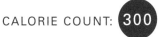 300

2 medium eggs
1 medium tomato, diced
Salt and pepper
Spray oil
1 ounce/30g grated Swiss cheese
A large handful of arugula leaves

Beat the eggs. Stir in the tomato and season with salt and pepper. Spray your pan and heat over low heat. Pour in the eggs and cook till just set. Top with the cheese and broil for 3 to 4 minutes to melt. Serve topped with arugula.

GRAVLAX WITH EGGS

CALORIE COUNT: 225

A classic smoked-fish-and-eggs combo. You could serve the eggs with a sprinkle of celery salt. You might like to keep a few hard-boiled eggs in the fridge to chaperone you through any hungry moments in the day.

3 ounces/85g gravlax or smoked salmon
1 medium egg, hard-boiled and peeled
A sprinkle of celery salt (optional)

Place gravlax on a plate and garnish with quartered egg. Season with celery salt, if using.

CRAB AND ARTICHOKES

CALORIE COUNT: **226**

This quick recipe comes from the River Café, a very, very famous restaurant in London, by way of my sister-in-law Clara, who adapted the idea to suit her own busy schedule. A container of lump crabmeat is no bad thing to toss into your shopping cart: tasty, responsible, plentiful, and about 87 calories per 3½-ounce/100g serving.

3 raw baby artichokes
Grated juice and zest of 1 lemon
3½ ounces/100g crabmeat
1 teaspoon minced garlic
2 teaspoons minced chives
Salt and pepper
1½ teaspoons good-quality olive oil
3½ ounces/100g baby arugula leaves

Remove the tough outer leaves and slice the the artichokes as thin as possible. (A mandoline works well.) Toss with the lemon juice to prevent discoloration. Mix with the crab, garlic, chives, lemon zest, salt and pepper, olive oil, and a generous handful of arugula leaves. Serve right away.

NB

GLOBE ARTICHOKES CONTAIN PROBIOTIC SUBSTANCES THAT CAN HELP IMPROVE GUT HEALTH.

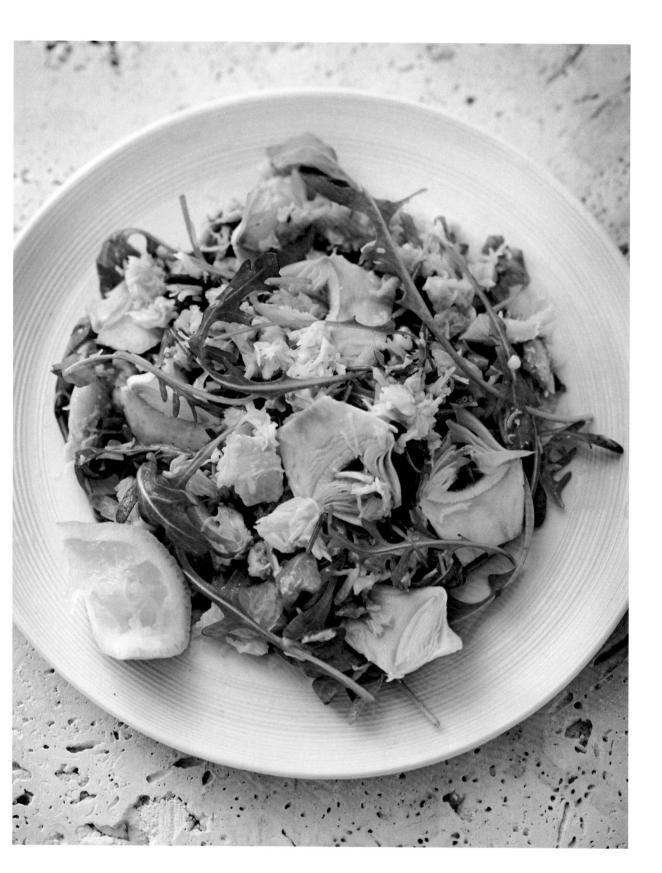

SUPER SIMPLE EGGPLANT CURRY

CALORIE COUNT:  298 WITH RICE 355

This must be the quickest curry this side of the Arabian Sea. There's something pleasing about its humble size and simplicity. But it really performs. Perhaps serve with a tablespoon of cooked brown rice mixed with 1 teaspoon cumin seed and topped with a scatter of flat-leaf parsley. You could also ditch the rice and add leafy vegetables to make it even more fast day–friendly.

1 small eggplant
1 tablespoon store-bought Indian curry paste
3 tablespoons/50ml vegetable stock
1 cup/200g unflavored low-fat yogurt
Chopped fresh cilantro

Preheat the oven to 400°F. Cut the eggplant in half lengthwise and score the inside quite deeply into cubes, leaving the skin intact, as you would a mango. Spread the cut surfaces with curry paste. Bake in an ovenproof skillet for 20 to 25 minutes, till the eggplant is soft. Remove from the oven and cut into cubes. Return to the pan and add the vegetable stock, yogurt, and cilantro. Stir to combine and cook till the sauce is heated through and a little thicker, about 10 minutes.

NB

EGGPLANTS SCORE A LOW 10 ON THE GI SCALE, AND JUST 0.5 ON GL.

RED PEPPER HUMMUS, CRUDITÉS, AND FLATBREAD DIPPERS

CALORIE COUNT: 256

Raw vegetable sticks are a no-brainer on a fast day. Hummus, meanwhile, scores an astonishing 0 on the GL score. It's relatively low in calories and high in fiber—a 2-tablespoon serving clocks in at about 46 calories (depending on type). Go for a light version to further improve the calorie cost. This is not so much a recipe as a loose collection of ingredients that work happily side by side. So play around and mix up your vegetables: pepper slices, broccoli florets, shredded white or red cabbage, jalapeños, some long, blushing French radishes? All welcome here.

2 tablespoons store-bought red pepper hummus (or flavor of your choice)
1 carrot, sliced into sticks
¼ garden cucumber or small seedless cucumber, sliced
1 stalk celery, cut into sticks
5 baby bell peppers, seeded and sliced
1 whole-grain pita, cut into strips and toasted
1 tablespoon Tahini Dip (optional)

Tahini dip

CALORIE COUNT FOR 1 TABLESPOON: 45

3 tablespoons/50ml unflavored low-fat yogurt
1 teaspoon lemon juice
1 teaspoon tahini
Chopped fresh mint

Mix well.

NB

HUMMUS IS A GOOD SOURCE OF VITAMIN E, A KEY ANTIOXIDANT.

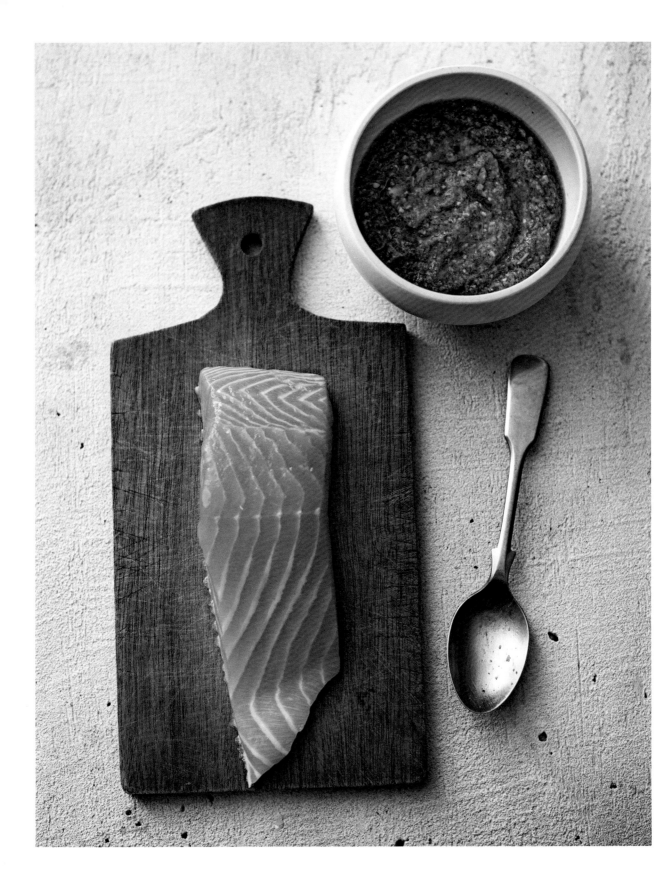

PESTO PRONTO SALMON WITH RIBBON VEGGIES

CALORIE COUNT: 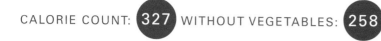 **327** WITHOUT VEGETABLES: **258**

A fast, fast fast day supper. Choose your salmon well: Tank-farmed salmon may be your best bet, given that wild Atlantic salmon stocks have been severely depleted, making them not only unsustainable, but expensive and hard to source.

3½ ounces/100g salmon fillet
1 tablespoon pesto, store-bought or homemade (page 210)
1 zucchini, cut lengthwise in ribbons with a vegetable peeler
1 red bell pepper, cut in strips
Spray oil

Preheat the broiler to medium, 350°F. Smear the salmon fillet with the pesto. Broil till the fish is cooked through, 15 to 20 minutes. Spray the zucchini ribbons and red bell pepper strips with a little oil. Place under the broiler with the fish for the final 6 minutes of cooking, turning halfway through. Serve the fish on a bed of the soft, charred ribbon veggies.

NB

THIS SUPPER CONTAINS 23G FAT, BUT MOST OF IT IS THE HEALTHY TYPE (MONOUNSATURATES AND OMEGA-3S).

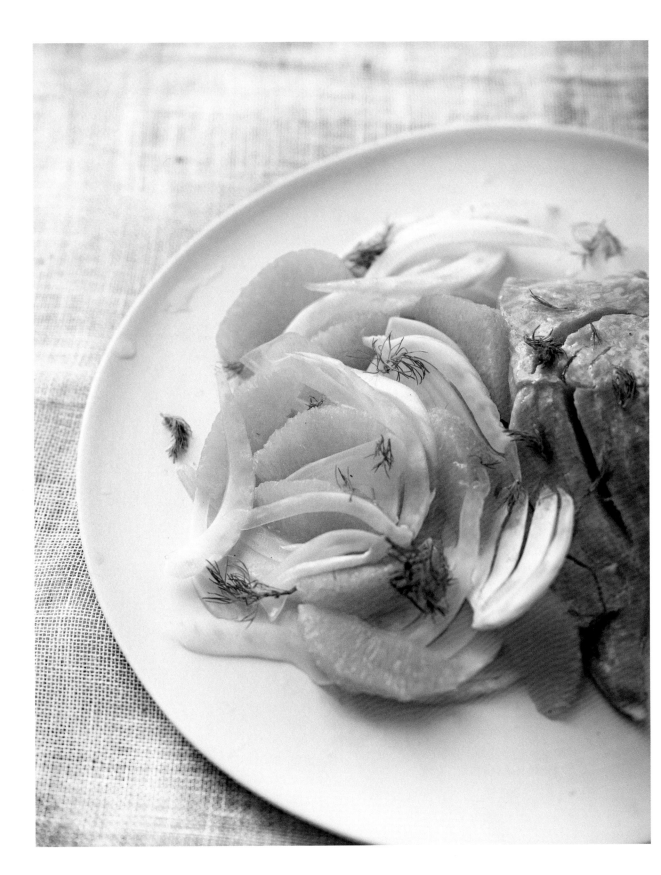

SALMON FOUR WAYS

CALORIE COUNT: 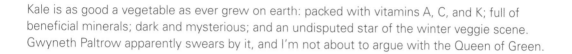 **180** FOR SALMON, PLUS ADDITIONAL FOR EXTRAS

Place a salmon fillet in a small baking pan, spray with oil, and bake at 350°F till the fish is cooked through, 15 to 20 minutes. Accompany . . .

With Peppered Kale

CALORIE COUNT: ADD **33**

Kale is as good a vegetable as ever grew on earth: packed with vitamins A, C, and K; full of beneficial minerals; dark and mysterious; and an undisputed star of the winter veggie scene. Gwyneth Paltrow apparently swears by it, and I'm not about to argue with the Queen of Green.

Steam 3½ ounces/100g curly kale over boiling water and pepper well before serving.

NB

KALE CONTAINS A SUBSTANCE CALLED INDOLE 3 CARBINOL, WHICH HAS BEEN SHOWN TO REPAIR DNA IN CELLS AND BLOCK THE GROWTH OF CANCER CELLS.[1]

With a Tangle of Steamed Samphire

CALORIE COUNT: ADD **49**

Samphire tastes of the sea, looks a picture, and is increasingly available at fishmongers and supermarkets such as Whole Foods, making it an ideal buddy for an ordinary salmon fillet.

Steam 3½ ounces/100g samphire lightly and introduce to a little lemon and a lot of pepper. Bliss.

NB

LIKE MANY SEA VEGETABLES, SAMPHIRE IS GOOD SOURCE OF IODINE, WHICH HELPS TO REGULATE THYROID HORMONES.

With a Shaved Fennel and Orange Salad

CALORIE COUNT: ADD 72

Fennel and orange have long been firm friends, so bring them together here to give a plain salmon fillet more than a bit on the side: crunch, color, and all-round good vibes.

Shave 1 bulb fennel (a mandoline works well) and combine with 1 orange, peeled and segmented, and its juice. Garnish with chopped fennel fronds.

NB

FENNEL CONTAINS ANETHOLE—A SUBSTANCE WITH ANTIOXIDANT AND ANTI-INFLAMMATORY PROPERTIES.[2]

With a Warm Puy Lentil Salad

CALORIE COUNT: ADD 195

Puy lentils are classic with salmon, but you can use brown, green, or any color you like.

Cover 1½ ounces/40g Puy lentils with cold water and add ½ chicken or vegetable bouillon cube. Simmer till tender, then drain. Toss together 3 halved cherry tomatoes, 1 ounce/30g minced red onion, ½ teaspoon minced garlic, 2 teaspoons lemon juice, 2 teaspoons olive oil, and chopped cilantro, plus salt and pepper. Stir through the cooling lentils and serve with the salmon. For a glorified version of this salad, see page 49.

SMOKED TROUT AND CELERY ROOT WITH HORSERADISH CREAM

CALORIE COUNT: **206**

The combination of ingredients here makes for a true taste-and-texture sensation—and, with a little preplanning, it's something you can haul from the fridge on a day when you're pressed for time. The smoked trout delivers a welcome jolt of omega-3 oils, and it's an attractive dish, too. One for a summer's evening.

2¼ ounces/60g watercress
Scant 2 ounces/50g celery root, thinly sliced
3½ ounces/100g smoked trout
Juice of ½ lemon
1 tablespoon crème fraîche or fromage blanc
1 teaspoon finely grated fresh horseradish

Place the watercress and celery root on a plate and flake the trout on top. Dress with lemon juice and a mix of crème fraîche and horseradish.

NB

AIM TO EAT PLENTY OF OILY FISH—THIS SMOKED TROUT WILL COUNT AS ONE OF YOUR WEEKLY PORTIONS.

COUSCOUS WITH LEMON AND MIRIN TOFU

CALORIE COUNT: 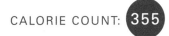 355

This is a complete and filling bowl of food—easy to prepare and attractive, to boot. The couscous here brings an added dimension, but if you make it with bulgur wheat instead of couscous, your GI and GL scores will fall.

Scant 2 ounces/50g instant couscous
3 tablespoons/50ml boiling water
1 teaspoon lemon juice
1 teaspoon mirin
2 scallions (green onions), sliced on the diagonal
3 cherry tomatoes, quartered
1 small zucchini, finely chopped
2 tablespoons/20g pine nuts
1 teaspoon sesame seeds
Salt and pepper
A handful of flat-leaf parsley, chopped
3 ounces/75g ready-marinated tofu

Place the couscous in a bowl and add the boiling water. Cover and set aside for 5 minutes. When ready, fork through and add the remaining ingredients, tofu last, and fold gently.

NB

THIS SUPPER PROVIDES NEARLY HALF A WOMAN'S RECOMMENDED DAILY AMOUNT OF IRON.

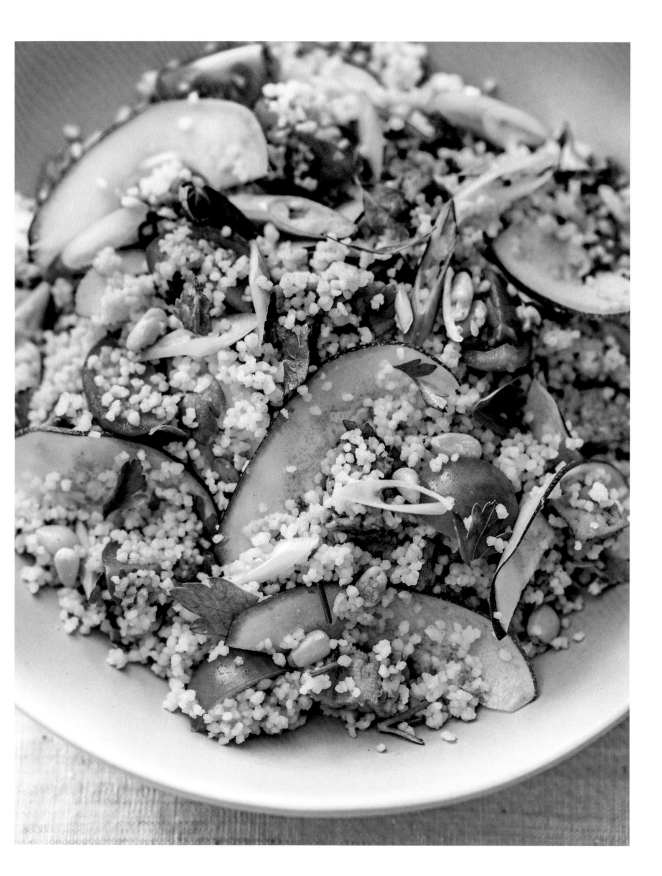

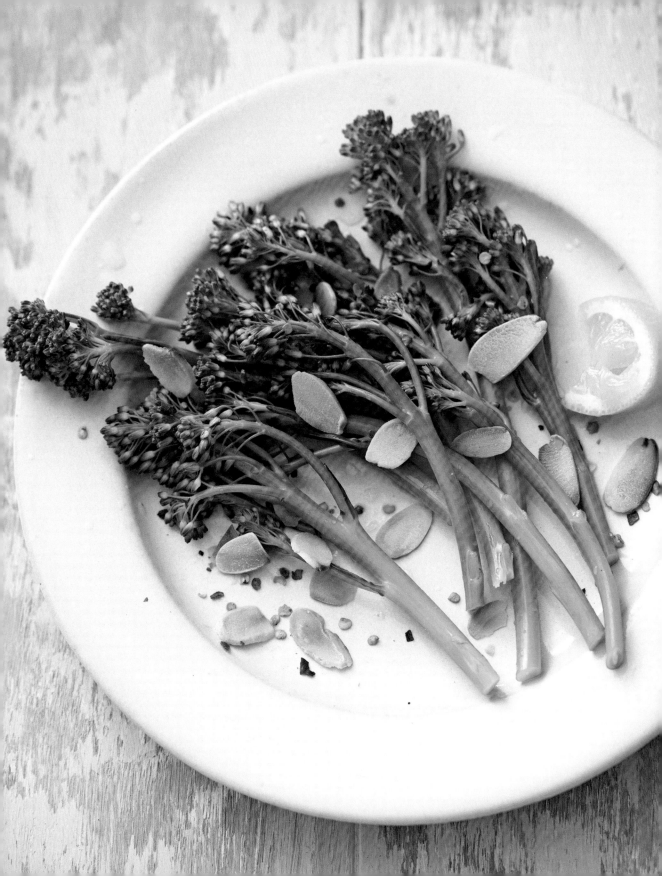

CHAPTER SEVEN

vegetables

BROCCOLI THREE WAYS

Broccoli is one of the most nutritious vegetables we know, rich in vitamins, folate, minerals (enough calcium to match most dairy products), iron, and fiber. And with a little imagination and not much effort on fast day, you can turn a head of broccoli into a superb supper.

Stir-Fried with Ginger, Garlic, Soy, and Hazelnuts

CALORIE COUNT: 132

Quickly blanch 3½ ounces/100g broccoli florets in boiling water, refresh in cold water, and drain. Heat a wok with 1 teaspoon peanut oil. Lightly stir-fry 1 teaspoon grated ginger and 1 teaspoon minced garlic, add blanched broccoli florets and red pepper, cooking till the broccoli is hot but not mushy. Serve topped with 1 tablespoon/10g chopped hazelnuts, flakes of sea salt, and a splash of soy sauce (½ teaspoon). This works wonderfully with steamed thin green beans, too.

Steamed Broccolini with Chili, Lemon, and Almonds

CALORIE COUNT: 157

Steam 3½ ounces/100g broccolini to your liking and dress with a squeeze of lemon, a pinch of red pepper flakes, and 2 tablespoons/20g toasted sliced almonds.

Broccoli Rabe with Bagna Cauda

CALORIE COUNT FOR THE BROCCOLI: **100** FOR 1 TABLESPOON

BAGNA CAUDA **85**

Blanch 10 ounces/300g broccoli rabe for 3 minutes, refresh in cold water, and drain. Place in a bowl with ½ teaspoon red pepper flakes, 1½ teaspoons good-quality olive oil, and 1 tablespoon lemon juice. Season with salt and pepper and serve drizzled with bagna cauda (page 84). For a simple alternative, serve steamed broccoli rabe with a finely chopped anchovy fillet, chopped olives, red pepper flakes, and a squeeze of lemon.

NB

BROCCOLI IS A FINE SOURCE OF VITAMIN K—IMPORTANT FOR BONE HEALTH.

CALABAZA CON ACELGAS

Pumpkin with Rainbow Chard and Wild Mushrooms

CALORIE COUNT: 133

A Mexican-style dish that ticks all the fast day boxes, delivering a great cargo of vegetables blessed with tons of flavor. Try it with other kinds of squash—butternut and pattypan spring to mind.

Serves 2

14 ounces/400g winter squash, seeded
1½ teaspoons olive oil
Salt and pepper
½ teaspoon dried oregano
½ teaspoon ground cumin
½ red onion, diced
1 clove garlic, minced
1 teaspoon finely chopped fresh chile
3 ounces/75g fresh wild mushrooms, chopped
3½ ounces/100g rainbow chard, leaves and stems, coarsely chopped
1½ tablespoons/20g pumpkin seeds (pepitas), toasted
A handful of fresh cilantro

Preheat the oven to 350°F. Cut the squash into wedges and place in a roasting pan. Drizzle with a little of the olive oil, salt, pepper, the oregano, and cumin. Roast for 30 minutes or till softened. While the squash is roasting, heat the remaining oil and cook the onion, garlic, and chile till tender. Add the mushrooms and cook till softened. Add the chard and cook for 5 to 6 minutes. Serve spiced pumpkin wedges with the chard mixture, a scatter of pumpkin seeds, and fresh cilantro.

NB

YELLOW-FLESH WINTER SQUASH ARE FULL OF VITAMIN A IN THE FORM OF BETA-CAROTENE AND OTHER CAROTENOIDS THAT HELP PREVENT OXIDATIVE DAMAGE TO CELLS IN THE BODY.

CHILE CHARD AND CHICKPEAS WITH ROASTED GARLIC

CALORIE COUNT: 145

For some reason, chard gets a hard time in the vegetable chart—which is a shame because it is abundant, inexpensive, and fantastically healthy. The chickpeas here will give you a punch of protein, while the chile lends a further kick. And the garlic? Don't leave out the garlic, which becomes sweet, sticky, and succulent in the oven (it loses its aftertaste too).

Serves 2

2 whole heads garlic, plus 1 clove, chopped
1 teaspoon olive oil
7 ounces/200g Swiss chard, stems removed and chopped, leaves sliced into fine ribbons
Salt and pepper
1 scallion (green onion), finely chopped
½ teaspoon ground cumin
1 red chile, thinly sliced
7 ounces/200g canned chickpeas, drained and rinsed
1 teaspoon lemon juice
A grating of lemon zest
A pinch of saffron threads
½ teaspoon paprika

Preheat the oven to 350°F. Wrap the whole heads of garlic in foil and roast till sweet and sticky, 25 to 30 minutes. You can do this a little in advance. Heat the oil in a large pan or wok. Stir-fry the chard stems. Season, then add the leaves. Cook till wilted and allow to cool on a side plate. Add the chopped garlic, scallion, cumin, and chile to the same pan. Stir-fry for a minute, then add the chickpeas, lemon juice and zest, saffron, and paprika. Return the chard to the pan and mix well, being sure to include any stickiness at the bottom of the pan. Serve with a head of sweet, soft garlic.

NB

CHARD IS HIGH IN VITAMINS A, C, AND K. VITAMIN K IS NEEDED TO HELP BLOOD CLOT NORMALLY.

SPICY EDAMAME

CALORIE COUNT: 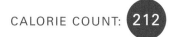 212

These green soybeans are a decent source of plant protein, fiber, and a host of vitamins and minerals. Try this recipe as a delicious dish to spoon alongside lean meat or fish.

Serves 2

1 tablespoon olive oil
2 shallots, thinly sliced
1 teaspoon grated fresh ginger
1 teaspoon garam masala or curry powder
½ teaspoon red pepper flakes
7 ounces/200g canned diced tomatoes
Salt and pepper
7 ounces/200g fresh or frozen edamame, shelled

Heat the olive oil and sauté the shallots. Add the ginger, garam masala, and red pepper. Stir, then add the tomatoes. Cook for 5 minutes, till the sauce has reduced. Season, add the edamame, and heat through.

NB

EDAMAME CONTAINS A GOOD BALANCE OF HEALTHY FATS, INCLUDING OMEGA-3S.

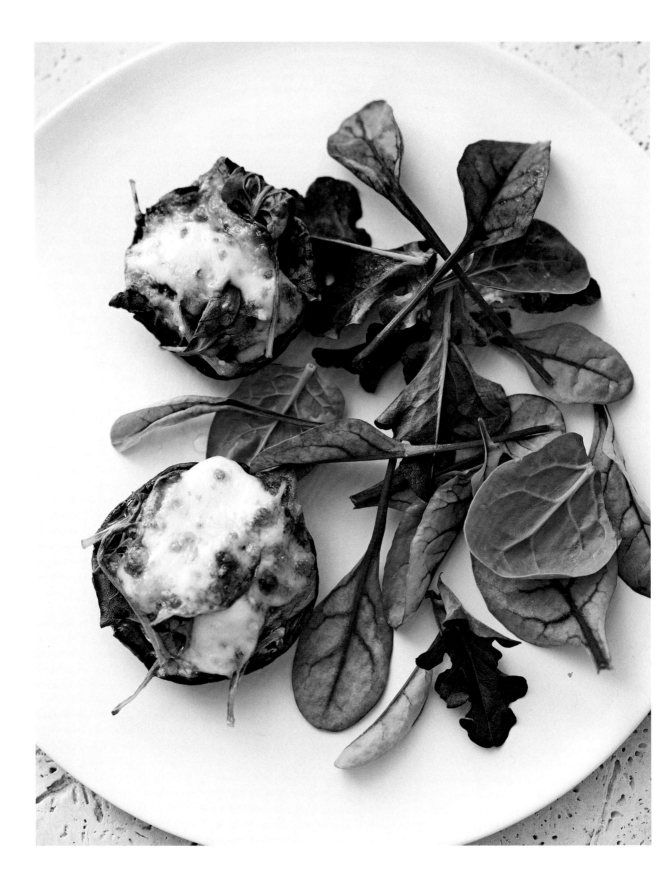

MUSHROOMS WITH MOZZARELLA, PECORINO, AND SPINACH

CALORIE COUNT: 159

Mushrooms are a good low-calorie substitute for beef,[1] so swap them when you can. This recipe works brilliantly as a breakfast, too, and makes good use of spinach, that unmatched fast day champion. If you can add spinach to your plate, always do.

3½ ounces/100g baby spinach leaves, blanched and refreshed
½ teaspoon red pepper flakes
1 teaspoon minced garlic
1 large or 2 medium white mushroom caps, wiped clean
Scant 2 ounces/50g low-fat mozzarella
2 teaspoons grated pecorino cheese
Fresh thyme leaves
Salt and pepper
Dressed salad leaves, for serving

Heat the broiler to 400°F. Mix the spinach, red pepper, and garlic in a small bowl and fill the mushrooms. Place the mushrooms on a slotted broiler pan and dot with the mozzarella. Scatter with the pecorino and thyme leaves and season. Broil for 7 to 10 minutes, till the cheese has melted and the mushrooms are cooked but still firm. Serve with a handful of dressed salad leaves.

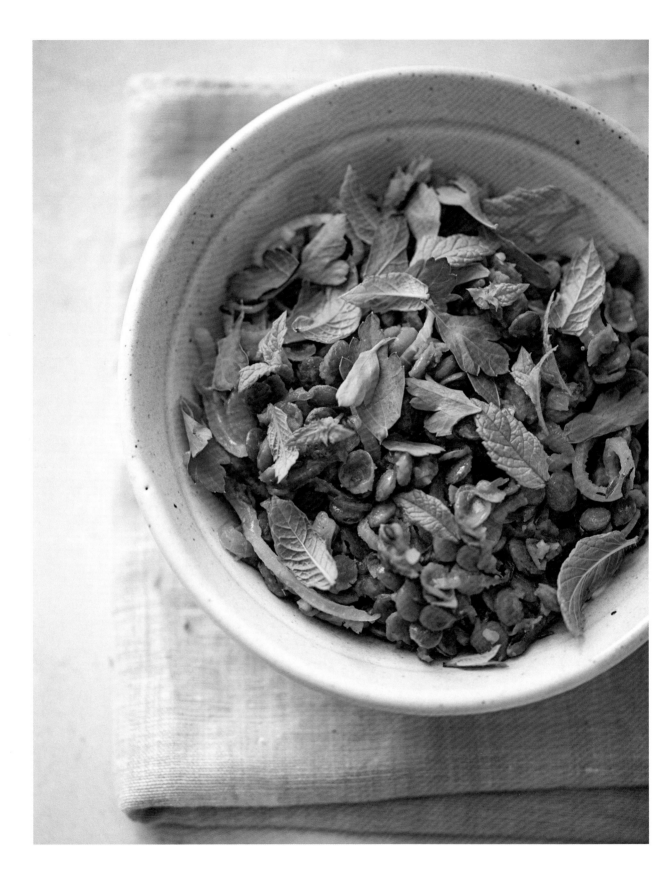

DAHL FOUR WAYS

Small but mighty, lentils (known generally as dahl throughout South Asia) are the little emperors of the veggie world. They pack protein and soluble fiber all the way, which means they have great satiating properties and an impressive capacity to help stabilize blood sugar. Dahl, then, is dynamite on a fast day, or any day, so here are four great ways to go with lentils.

All dahls can be loosened with vegetable stock to make a soup that is nutritious and heartwarming (a study published in the *Archives of Internal Medicine* confirms that eating high-fiber foods such as lentils helps prevent heart disease).[2]

Red Tomato Dahl

CALORIE COUNT: **190**

Serves 2

½ teaspoon flaxseed oil
1 red onion, thinly sliced
¼ teaspoon ground turmeric
½ teaspoon ground cumin
½ teaspoon black mustard seeds
A pinch of red pepper flakes
1 clove garlic, chopped
1 pound/500g tomatoes, peeled and coarsely chopped
3 ounces/75g red lentils, rinsed
2½ cups/600ml water
Salt and pepper
A handful of fresh cilantro leaves, chopped
Diced fresh tomato and scallion (green onion), for serving

Heat the oil in a saucepan. Add the onion and cook till soft and slightly browned. Stir in the turmeric, cumin, mustard seeds, and red pepper and cook gently for another minute. Add the garlic, chopped tomatoes, and lentils. Stir in the water and simmer for 30 minutes, adding more water if necessary to achieve the desired consistency and prevent sticking. Season and serve with cilantro, diced tomato, and diced scallion.

NB

OVER 4G OF FIBER PER SERVING PROVIDES A QUARTER OF YOUR RECOMMENDED DAILY INTAKE.

Green Lentils and Mint

CALORIE COUNT: 224

Serves 4

9 ounce/250g green lentils, rinsed
3½ cups/800ml cold water
1 teaspoon ground turmeric
1 tablespoon sunflower oil
1 teaspoon cumin seeds
1 white onion, thinly sliced
Salt and pepper
Fresh mint and parsley leaves, for serving

Put the lentils in a pan with the water and bring to a boil. Skim off froth, then stir in the turmeric. Reduce the heat and simmer, uncovered, for 15 to 20 minutes, stirring occasionally, till soft. Add a little boiling water if too thick. Heat the oil in a small pan and cook the cumin seeds for a minute, then add the onion and sauté for 5 minutes, till softened. Add the onion mix to the cooked lentils. Season and serve topped with plenty of mint and parsley.

NB

EVEN MORE FIBER—7G PER PORTION.

Yellow Tarka Dahl

CALORIE COUNT: 237

Serves 4

9 ounces/250g dried split chickpeas, rinsed
1 quart plus scant ½ cup/1.1 liters water
1 tablespoon sunflower oil
1 tablespoon cumin seeds
1 small onion, diced
3 whole green chiles, slit
¾-inch piece fresh ginger, peeled and
    julienned

3 whole peeled cloves garlic
3 tomatoes
½ teaspoon ground turmeric
1 teaspoon garam masala or curry powder
1 teaspoon ground coriander
Salt and pepper
A handful of fresh parsley, chopped, for
    serving

Place the chickpeas and 1 quart water in a pan, stir, and bring to a boil. Skim off any froth. Cover and reduce the heat. Simmer, stirring regularly, for 35 to 40 minutes, or till the chickpeas are just tender, adding more water as necessary. Set aside. Heat the oil in a pan over medium heat. Add cumin seeds and cook for 20 to 30 seconds, then add the onion, chiles, and ginger and sauté for 4 to 5 minutes, till golden brown. Puree the garlic and tomatoes in a food processor and add to the pan, stirring well to combine. Add the ground spices and ½ cup water and stir well to combine. Season and simmer for 15 minutes, then skim any oil from the surface. Stir the cooked chickpeas into the sauce, adding more water to loosen if necessary. Heat through and serve with plenty of chopped parsley.

NB

THIS RECIPE ALSO HAS 7G FIBER.

Spinach, Pea, and Lime Dahl

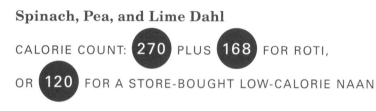

CALORIE COUNT: 270 PLUS 168 FOR ROTI,

OR 120 FOR A STORE-BOUGHT LOW-CALORIE NAAN

Serves 4

1 tablespoon peanut oil
1 large onion, diced
4 cloves garlic, minced
1 red chile, finely chopped
2 teaspoons grated fresh ginger
½ teaspoon ground turmeric
½ teaspoon cayenne pepper
1 teaspoon paprika

9 ounces/250g red lentils, rinsed
2½ cups/600ml water
2 ripe tomatoes, peeled and coarsely
   chopped
3 tablespoons frozen peas
A handful of baby spinach leaves
Juice of 1 lime
Salt and pepper

Gently heat the oil in a large pan and add the onion, garlic, chile, and ginger. Sauté for 5 minutes, till softened. Add the spices and cook for 2 minutes more. Add the lentils and stir to coat in the onion-spice mixture. Add the water, stir, and bring to a boil. Reduce heat to a simmer and cook for 30 minutes, stirring occasionally so that dahl does not stick, adding more water if it becomes too thick. Stir in the tomatoes, peas, spinach, and lime juice. Season and serve with Rye Barley Roti (page 88) or a low-calorie naan bread.

NB

THERE IS 6G FIBER PER PORTION IN THIS RECIPE.

BAGNA CAUDA WITH GRILLED VEGETABLES

CALORIE COUNT PER TABLESPOON BAGNA CAUDA: **85**

CALORIE COUNT WITH GRILLED VEGETABLES: ABOUT **205**

This centuries-old Piedmontese sauce is cooked slowly—some might say lovingly—to develop its earthy, pungent flavors. Bagna cauda means "hot bath," and that's really what your grilled veggies will be getting. Bagna cauda is robust (and calorific), but a little goes a long way, as is the case with anything that involves anchovy. Ricotta is good on the side, and a handful of pine nuts would be welcome too, calories permitting.

Makes about 1½ cups/350ml sauce, 24 servings

Bagna cauda
1 tablespoon butter
15 large cloves garlic, minced
3½ ounces/100g flat anchovy fillets,
    drained and oil reserved, minced
Scant ½ cup/100ml olive oil
1½ cups/350ml whole milk
Cracked black pepper

Grilled vegetables
Eggplant, thickly sliced
Cauliflower florets, blanched
Broccoli florets, blanched
Red and yellow bell peppers, cut in wide
    strips

Fennel bulb, quartered
Leeks, washed and cut into chunks
Radicchio, quartered
Endive, halved lengthwise
Portobello mushrooms, thickly sliced
Zucchini, halved lengthwise
Onions, quartered
Whole head garlic
Spray olive oil
Salt and pepper
Asparagus, blanched
Mixed fresh herbs leaves, for serving

For the bagna cauda: Melt the butter in a heavy saucepan over medium heat. Add the minced garlic and sauté, stirring constantly, for 30 seconds. Reduce the heat to low and cook, stirring, for about 5 minutes. Add the anchovies and their oil and cook, stirring, for 2 minutes. Add the olive oil and cook till the anchovy-garlic mixture is golden brown, about 8 minutes. Do not let it burn. Add the milk. Bring to a boil, reduce the heat to very low, and simmer, whisking occasionally, for 20 minutes. Season generously with pepper. Whisk vigorously to stabilize the emulsion. Pour the sauce into a heatproof container.

Meanwhile, roast or grill the vegetables, sprayed with olive oil and seasoned, for 20 minutes, adding the asparagus for the final 10 minutes. Serve each portion with a tablespoon of bagna cauda spooned over it and topped with fresh herb leaves. It's meant to look rustic and improvised, so don't be too particular.

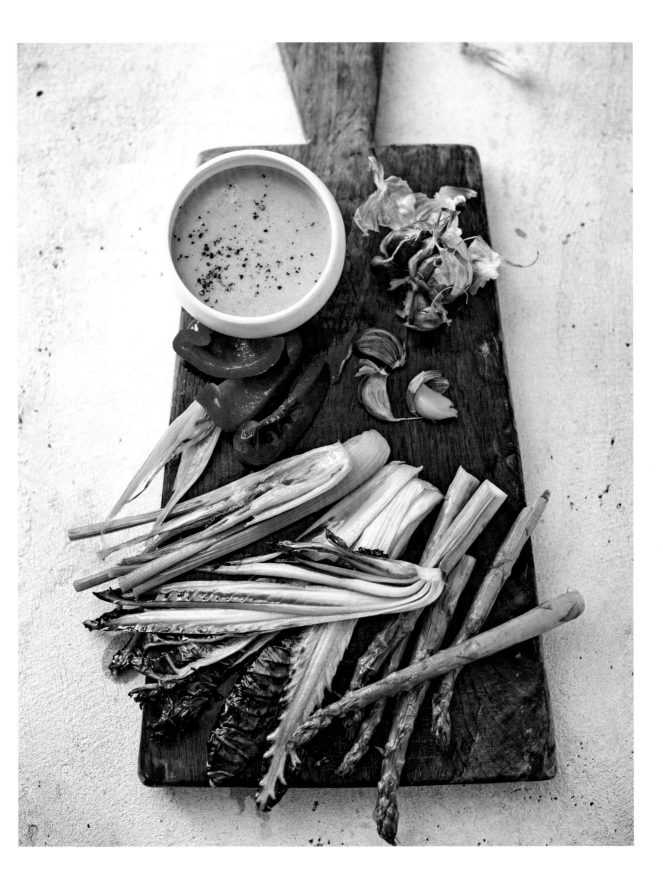

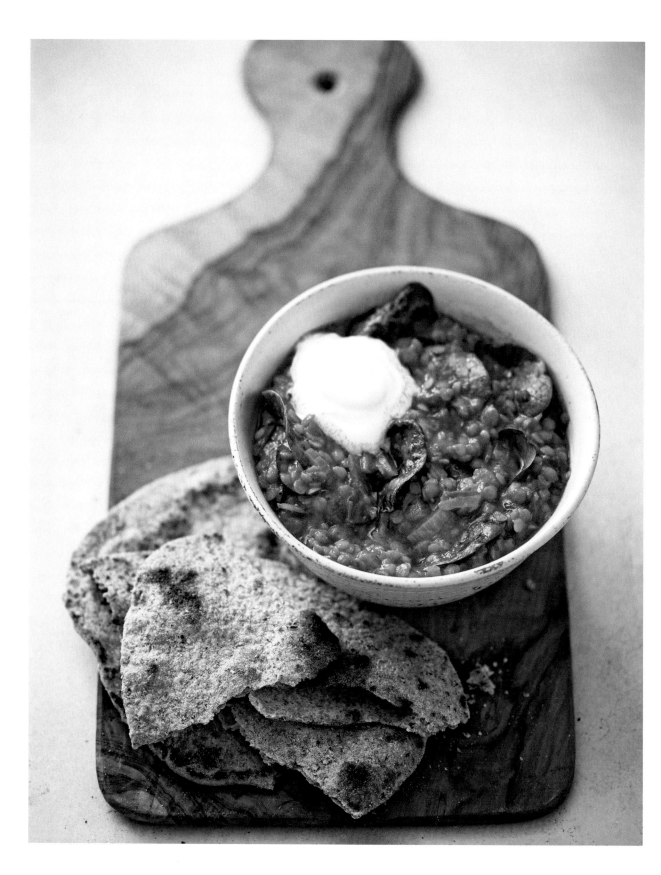

RED LENTIL TIKKA MASALA WITH
RYE BARLEY ROTI

CALORIE COUNT: 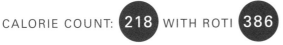 218 WITH ROTI 386

Utterly delicious and authentically spicy. Really, who needs chicken? You may not need the roti either—though it's a great bonus if you can spare the calories.

Serves 4

Masala paste
2 teaspoons garam masala or curry powder
2 teaspoons red pepper flakes
2 teaspoons smoked paprika
1 teaspoon cumin seeds, toasted and ground
1 teaspoon coriander seed, toasted and ground
¾-inch piece fresh ginger, peeled and grated
1 tablespoon peanut oil
2 tablespoons tomato paste
Salt and pepper
A handful of fresh cilantro

Curry
1½ tablespoons peanut oil
1 red onion, diced
1 clove garlic, minced
2 tablespoons masala paste (from above)
One 14-ounce/400g can diced tomatoes
1 cup/250ml vegetable stock
7 ounces/200g red lentils, rinsed
7 ounces/200g baby spinach leaves

2 tablespoons unflavored low-fat yogurt
Rye Barley Roti (recipe follows), for serving

Pulse the masala paste ingredients in a mini food processor till well combined and fairly smooth. (Store any extra in a covered container in the fridge.) For the curry, heat the oil in a large skillet, add the onion, and cook till softened, 3 to 4 minutes. Add the garlic and cook for 1 minute more. Stir in the masala paste and cook to release flavors, then add the tomatoes and stock and bring to a boil. Add the lentils, reduce the heat, and simmer for 20 minutes. Remove from the heat and add the spinach leaves, allowing them to wilt in the warmth. If necessary, loosen with a little more hot stock. Serve with a dollop of yogurt and a warm rye barley roti.

NB

OIL IS LIMITED HERE; THE FLAVORS COME INSTEAD FROM A HOST OF VIBRANT SPICES.

Rye Barley Roti

3½ ounces/100g whole wheat flour, scant 2 ounces/50g barley flour, and scant 2 ounces/50g rye flour,
    or 7 ounces/200g whole wheat flour
½ teaspoon coarse sea salt
A pinch of chili powder
1 teaspoon cumin seeds
½ teaspoon caraway seeds
1 teaspoon olive oil
½ cup/120ml water
Spray oil

Mix all the ingredients and knead to a smooth dough. Allow to rest for 20 minutes. Knead well and divide into 8 balls. Roll each ball into a disk, using a little more whole wheat flour to prevent sticking. Spray a heavy skillet with a hint of oil and cook the breads on both sides till cooked through.

WILD MUSHROOMS WITH SAGE, SOFT POACHED EGG, AND PARMESAN

CALORIE COUNT: 236

For me, wild mushrooms still feel like a mystical treat, with their flavor of the deep woods. Combined with downy sage, a yielding egg, and the salt-tang of Parmesan, they make a heavenly plate of food.

1 ounce/30g dried porcini mushrooms
1 teaspoon olive oil
1 small red chile, finely chopped
½ teaspoon minced garlic
2 fresh sage leaves, plus more for serving
3½ ounces/100g wild mushrooms, any type, washed and dried
Salt and pepper
1 medium egg
Scant 2 ounces/50g arugula leaves
A shaving of Parmesan cheese (about 1 teaspoon)

Cover the porcini with boiling water and let soak till softened, 10 minutes. Lift out of the water, chop, and set aside. Strain the liquor through a coffee filter and set aside. Heat the oil in a skillet and gently cook the chile, garlic, and sage for 2 minutes. Add the wild mushrooms, the porcini, and their liquor. Cook for a minute or so and season. While the mushrooms are cooking, poach the egg in a large pan of salted boiling water (see page 14). Combine the warm mushroom mix with the arugula leaves and top with the egg. Add a shaving of Parmesan and torn fresh sage leaves to serve.

NB

WILD MUSHROOMS OFTEN CONTAIN MORE SELENIUM THAN CULTIVATED MUSHROOMS, AS THEY MAY HAVE GROWN IN MINERAL-RICH SOIL.

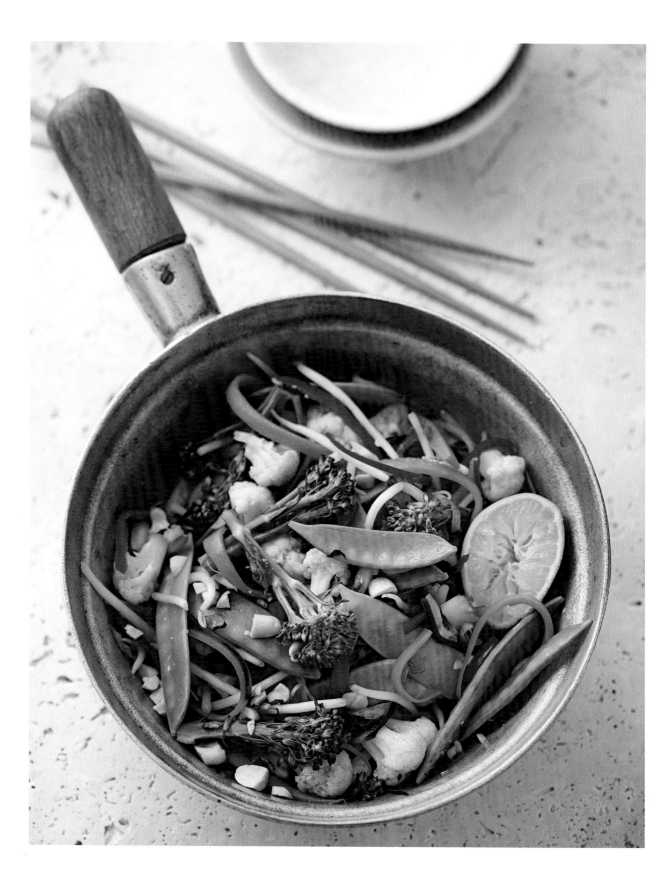

HOT THAI STIR-FRY

CALORIE COUNT: **229** WITH PEANUTS **341**

Here's another opportunity to go wild with the greens and consume as many vegetables as you can usefully fit into one sitting. You could eat, say, bean sprouts as a panda does bamboo and never really put on any weight (they're about 30 calories per 3½ ounces/100g, which is virtually nothing). The trio of fish sauce, soy sauce, and lime juice, plus ginger and chile, is a total Thai classic and works brilliantly here to deliver supercharged zing.

1 tablespoon peanut oil
2¼ ounces/60g red cabbage, thinly sliced or shredded
1 small red onion, thinly sliced
1 carrot, julienned
2¼ ounces/60g cauliflower florets, chopped
2¼ ounces/60g broccoli florets, chopped
1 ounce/30g snow peas
1 ounce/30g bean sprouts, plus more for serving
1 clove garlic, minced
½ red chile, thinly sliced
1 teaspoon grated fresh ginger
½ teaspoon coriander seeds
1 tablespoon soy sauce
1 teaspoon Asian fish sauce
A squeeze of lime juice
10 unsalted peanuts, chopped, for serving (optional)

Heat the oil in a wok on high. Add the vegetables in order and stir-fry for 3 minutes, then add the garlic, chile, ginger, and coriander and stir-fry for a few minutes more. Add the soy sauce, fish sauce, and lime juice for the final minute of cooking and serve with more raw bean sprouts, and chopped peanuts if your calorie count allows.

NB

KEEP THE VEGGIES CRUNCHY—IT CAN HELP RETAIN THEIR VITAMIN CONTENT.

TRIPLE BEAN STEW WITH VANILLA

CALORIE COUNT: 237

Lots of protein, loads of fiber, and plenty of vitamins for very few calories: Beans make sense on a fast day. Jazz them up with unusual flavors—if you can find it, add pandan leaf, with its smoky notes—but do have a go with the vanilla pod, a surprising and effective pairing that will turn any old bean stew into something altogether more interesting.

Serves 4

1 tablespoon peanut oil
2 shallots, finely chopped
1 small leek (white and pale green parts), thinly sliced and washed thoroughly
1 stalk celery, thinly sliced
½ bulb fennel, diced
28 ounces/800g mixed drained canned beans (small, light-colored beans are the best, perhaps navy beans and black-eyed peas)
½ pandan leaf, crushed (optional)
A pinch of red pepper flakes
1 bay leaf
Scant ½ cup/100ml vegetable stock
½ vanilla pod, split
Salt and pepper

Heat the oil in a large pan and add the shallots. Sauté for a minute, then add the leek, celery, and fennel. Sauté till softened. Add the beans, pandan leaf (if using), red pepper, bay leaf, and stock. Simmer for 10 to 15 minutes, allowing the stew to reduce a little. Add the seeds scraped from the vanilla pod. Season and serve with a steamed dark green leaf such as kale.

NB

LEGUMES SUCH AS BEANS PROVIDE VITAMIN B_6, IMPORTANT FOR CELLULAR FUNCTION AND BRAIN CHEMISTRY.

SHORBAT RUMMAN

Iraqi Pomegranate Stew

CALORIE COUNT: 410

On a cold winter's day, this will fill you up and warm your bones—a luscious alternative to the Indian curries we all know and love. The pomegranate molasses lends further depth (it's easily sourced in supermarkets).

Serves 2

2 teaspoons olive oil
1 large onion, diced
2 cloves garlic, crushed
1 cinnamon stick, broken
1 teaspoon ground cumin
½ teaspoon ground fenugreek
A pinch of saffron threads
3½ ounces/100g dried yellow split peas
1 vegetable bouillon cube
1 quart/1 liter vegetable stock

3½ ounces/100g brown basmati rice
A large handful of spinach, chopped
2 scallions (green onions), sliced
1 tablespoon lemon juice
1 tablespoon pomegranate molasses
Salt and pepper
A handful of fresh cilantro, chopped
A handful of fresh mint leaves, chopped
Pomegranate seeds, for garnish

Heat the oil in a large saucepan and sauté the onion till softened. Add the garlic and spices and cook for a few minutes more. Add the split peas, bouillon cube, and stock and simmer for 45 minutes or till just cooked, stirring occasionally to check that the stew is loose and not sticking (if it does stick, add more stock). Add the rice and cook for 20 to 25 minutes more, again watching the consistency. Stir in the spinach, scallions, lemon juice, pomegranate molasses, and salt and pepper. To serve, scatter with cilantro, mint, pomegranate seeds, and a final twist of cracked black pepper.

NB

SPLIT PEAS ARE LOW-GI AND WILL THICKEN THIS RICH STEW.

ROASTED VEGETABLES WITH SPICED BALSAMIC GLAZE

CALORIE COUNT 261 WITH GOAT CHEESE 309

This is a premium version of the simple roasted vegetables we endlessly sling into the oven with a "slug of olive oil." It amounts to a proper meal in itself, complete with sticky bits, gorgeous balsamic color, and bursts of spiced flavor. Personally, I'd include the goat cheese and save calories elsewhere; it's too good to miss.

Serves 2

½ teaspoon cumin seeds
½ teaspoon nigella seeds
½ teaspoon mustard seeds
1 tablespoon olive oil
1 red onion, sliced
3 cloves garlic, minced
½ red chile, finely chopped
1 red bell pepper, sliced
1 yellow bell pepper, sliced
1 orange bell pepper, sliced
1 zucchini, thickly sliced
1 small eggplant, thickly sliced
1 small butternut squash, unpeeled but cubed and seeded
Fresh marjoram leaves
Juice of 1 lemon
1 tablespoon good-quality balsamic vinegar
Green salad with lots of pepper, for serving
½ ounce/15g dry aged goat cheese (or manchego) and pickled guindilla peppers, for serving (optional)

Preheat the oven to 425°F. In a small skillet, gently toast the seeds, then add the oil and onion and cook till softened. Add the garlic and chile and cook for 2 minutes more. Place the vegetables in a roasting pan and stir in the spiced onion mix, marjoram, lemon juice, and vinegar, making sure that everything is well coated. Roast for 20 to 30 minutes, till caramelized and sticky. Serve with a peppery green salad plus a shaving of goat cheese or manchego and pickled guindillas, if you like.

NB

ALL THESE COLORS INDICATE PLENTY OF BETA-CAROTENE AND OTHER IMPORTANT ANTIOXIDANTS.

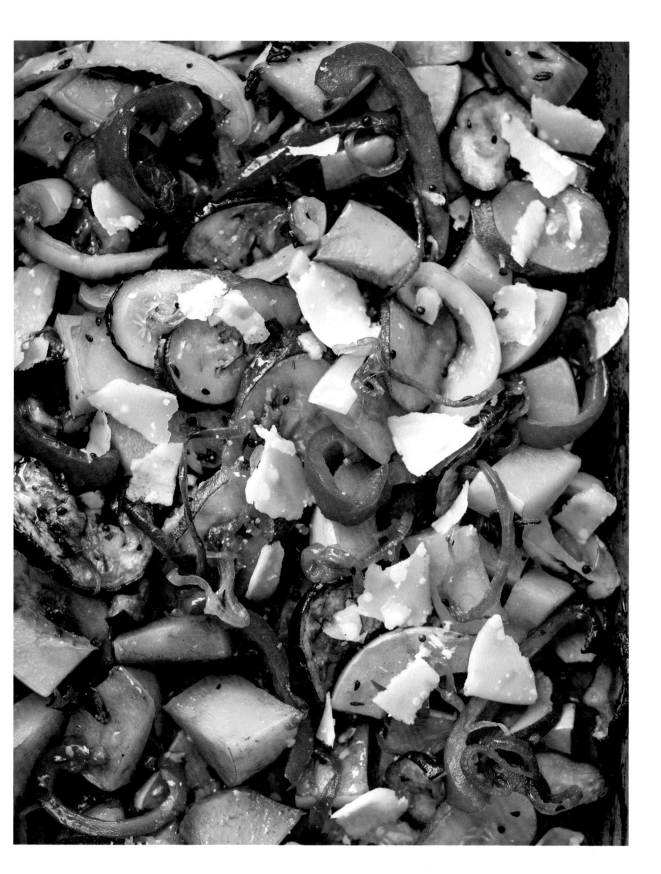

SPICED BABY EGGPLANT WITH POMEGRANATE YOGURT

CALORIE COUNT: 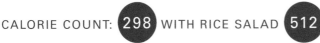 **298** WITH RICE SALAD **512**

No recipe book is complete these days without the obligatory pomegranate seeds scattered over anything that doesn't move—and here they bring a touch of ruby magic to a brilliantly balanced, terrifically appealing dish. The rice, though nice, will whack up the calorie count considerably, so include it only if your budget allows.

Serves 2

1 medium onion, chopped
1 tablespoon olive oil
1 clove garlic, minced
1 tablespoon grated fresh ginger
1 tablespoon harissa paste
2 teaspoons cumin seeds
2 teaspoons ground coriander
4 baby eggplants, halved lengthwise
One 14-ounce/400g can diced tomatoes
1 tablespoon tomato paste
A squeeze of lemon juice
½ teaspoon sugar
Salt and pepper
7 ounces/200g canned chickpeas, drained
A handful of fresh cilantro leaves
1 tablespoon unflavored low-fat yogurt
A handful of pomegranate seeds
Walnut–Brown Rice Salad (recipe follows), for serving (optional)

Soften the onion in the olive oil and add the garlic, ginger, harissa, cumin, and coriander. Cook for 3 minutes and add the eggplant, tomatoes, tomato paste, lemon juice, sugar, and salt and pepper. Simmer for 30 minutes. Add the chickpeas to heat through, plus a tablespoon of water if the sauce is too thick. Top with cilantro, drizzle with yogurt, scatter with pomegranate seeds, and serve with a side of nutty rice salad.

NB

POMEGRANATES CONTAIN ANTIOXIDANTS WITH THE POTENTIAL TO SCAVENGE FREE RADICALS THAT CAUSE DAMAGE TO BODY CELLS.

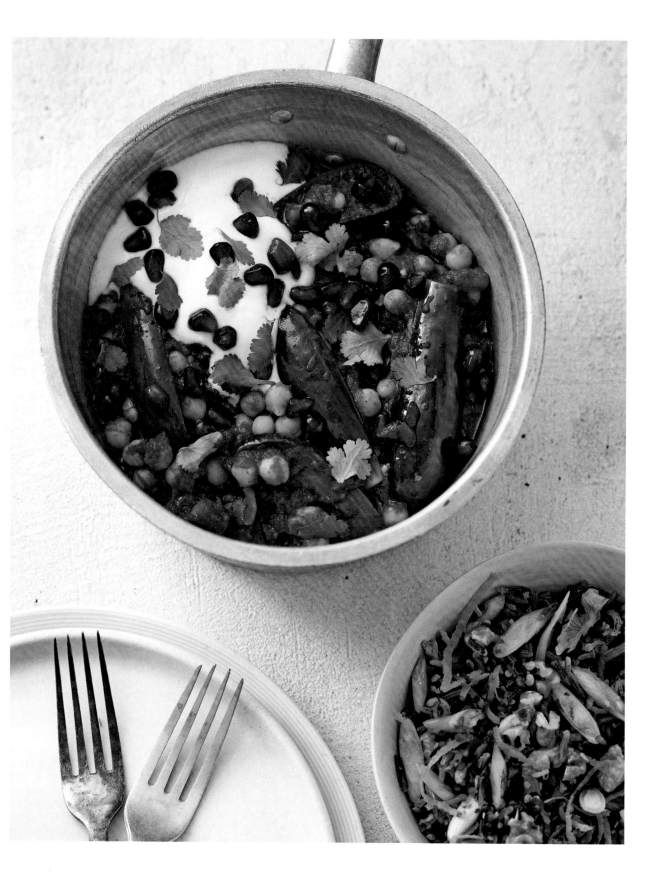

Walnut–Brown Rice Salad

Scant 2 ounces/50g brown rice, cooked till tender, drained and cooled
¾ ounce/20g walnuts, chopped
1 scallion (green onion), finely chopped
2 teaspoons orange zest curls
1 tablespoon orange juice
½ teaspoon red pepper flakes
Salt and pepper
Fresh cilantro leaves

Combine the ingredients, mix, and serve topped with cilantro.

RED VEGETABLE GOULASH WITH KOHLRABI AND RADISH SALAD

CALORIE COUNT: 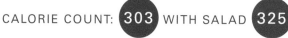 303 WITH SALAD 325

The paprika brings a smoky hum to the proceedings here, and again, this recipe gives you a whole world of vegetables in a bowl. Cut through the dense flavors with a crisp, crunchy salad. And fear not the humble kohlrabi—this knobbly cousin of the cabbage is worth seeking out: It is in fact enormously nutritious, stuffed with minerals and good old-fashioned vitamin C.

Serves 4

1 tablespoon peanut oil
2 medium red onions, chopped
1 clove garlic, halved
2 teaspoons Hungarian sweet paprika
1 teaspoon smoked paprika
2 teaspoons dried oregano
1 teaspoon dried basil
2 red bell peppers, sliced
2 carrots, thickly sliced
7 ounces/200g canned or frozen lima beans, drained and rinsed

3½ ounces/100g canned kidney beans, drained and rinsed
3½ ounces/100g red split lentils, rinsed
4 large ripe tomatoes, peeled and chopped
2 tablespoons tomato paste
3¼ cups/750ml vegetable stock
¾ cup/150ml red wine
1 whole dried chile (optional)
Salt and pepper
Kohlrabi and Radish Salad (recipe follows)

Heat the oil in a large heavy saucepan and sauté the onion till softened. Add the garlic and sauté for a minute more. Stir in the paprikas, oregano, and basil. Add the peppers and carrots and cook for 5 minutes more. Add the beans, lentils, tomatoes, tomato paste, stock, and wine. Place the dried chile in the broth, if using, and simmer for 20 minutes till the lentils are cooked through and the dish is thickened. Remove the chile, season the goulash, and serve with the salad.

NB

RADISHES CONTAIN A TYPE OF FIBER CALLED ARABINOGALACTAN, WHICH IS GOOD FOR BOOSTING FRIENDLY BACTERIA IN THE GUT.

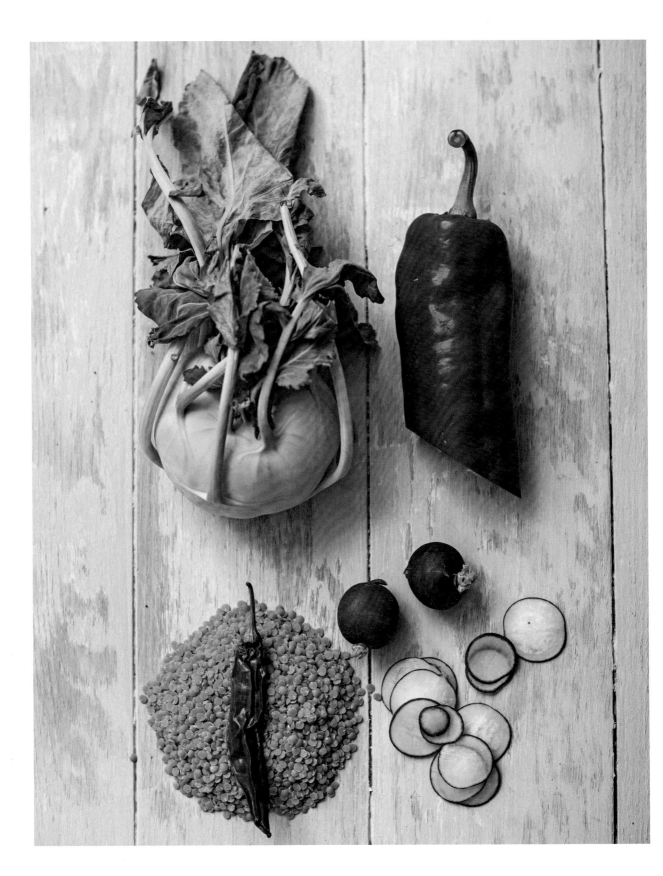

Kohlrabi and Radish Salad

Dress 2 large knobs kohlrabi, trimmed, peeled, and thinly sliced and a large handful of radishes, also thinly sliced, with a vinaigrette made from 2 teaspoons white wine vinegar, 1 teaspoon lime juice, 1 teaspoon peanut oil, 1 teaspoon poppy seeds, 1 teaspoon fennel seeds, and a pinch of sugar. Garnish with torn flat-leaf parsley.

HOT, SWEET, AND SOUR TOFU

CALORIE COUNT: 345

On its own, tofu is nothing special—in fact it's a bit of a bore. But marinate it and it springs to life, soaking up flavor and bringing fine low-fat protein to your fork. Use firm tofu; the silken variety is best for blending, while the firm should hold its shape in the wok. Firm tofu also tends to contain the most calcium. It should be pressed dry before cooking or marinating. Searing tofu, just as you would sear meat, blesses it with a golden exterior and the promise of a wobbling white interior, a fabulous foil to the al dente crunch of the peppers.

1½ teaspoons peanut oil

3½ ounces/100g firm tofu, cut into cubes or slices, press-dried on paper towels

1 clove garlic, minced

1 scallion (green onion), chopped

2 teaspoons grated fresh ginger

A pinch of red pepper flakes

Scant 2 ounces/50g red or yellow bell pepper, thinly sliced

Scant 2 ounces/50g cremini mushrooms, sliced

Scant 2 ounces/50g broccoli, blanched and refreshed

Scant 2 ounces/50g bean sprouts, plus more for garnish

1 tablespoon soy sauce

1 teaspoon agave nectar

A squeeze of lemon juice

Heat the oil in a wok. Stir-fry the tofu cubes till golden; gently transfer to paper towels. Put the wok back over medium heat and add the garlic, scallion, ginger, and red pepper, plus a tablespoon of water if they stick. Stir-fry for 2 minutes, then turn up the heat and add the vegetables in order. Add the soy sauce, agave nectar, and lemon juice. Cook for 4 to 5 minutes more, till the vegetables are just cooked but still firm. Return the tofu to the wok and gently stir through. Top with more raw bean sprouts to garnish.

NB

TOFU IS MADE FROM SOYBEANS, A LOW-FAT SOURCE OF "COMPLETE" PROTEIN, CONTAINING ALL NINE AMINO ACIDS ESSENTIAL FOR HUMAN NUTRITION.

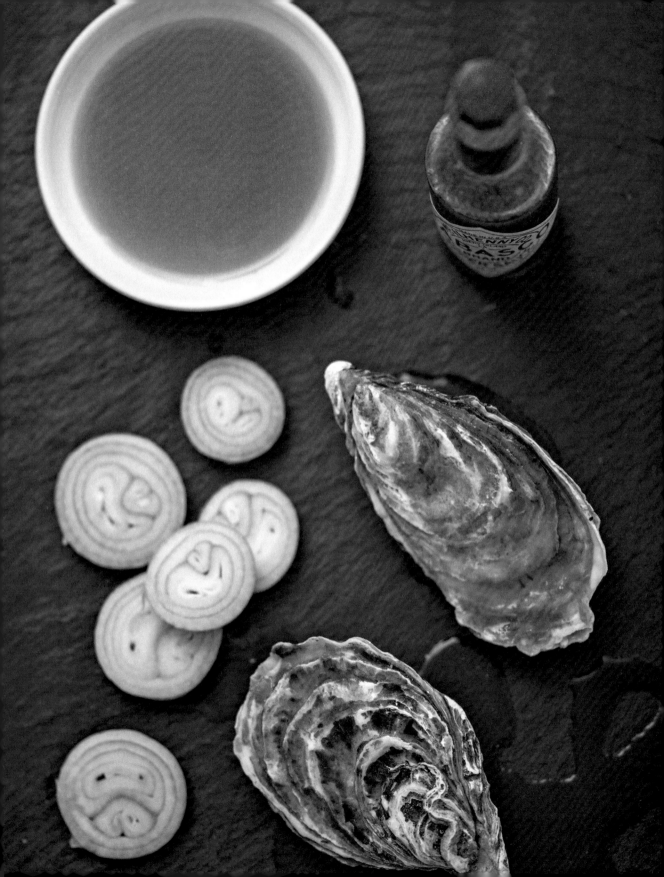

CHAPTER EIGHT

fish

OYSTERS WITH MIGNONETTE

CALORIE COUNT: 53

Oysters are thoroughly nutritious and healthy; stick to the September–April season and discard any oysters with shells that are open, cracked, or damaged. The traditional accompaniment is mignonette, which in rough translation means "cute, small, and tasty." Precisely.

Makes about ½ cup sauce

Mignonette

3 tablespoons/50ml white wine vinegar
3 tablespoons/50ml rice vinegar or red wine vinegar
2 or 3 small shallots, very finely minced
¼ teaspoon sugar
¼ teaspoon salt
1 teaspoon ground white pepper
Tabasco sauce (optional)

6 fresh oysters (per person), opened

Place the mignonette ingredients in a glass bowl and stir with a fork. Cover and chill for a minimum of 4 hours. You can make it a day ahead to allow the shallots to mellow in the acid of the vinegar. It will keep for 2 weeks or more in the fridge. Perhaps add a dash of Tabasco to taste. Serve with the oysters.

NB

OYSTERS ARE A GREAT SOURCE OF ZINC, WHICH BOOSTS THE IMMUNE SYSTEM, HEALS WOUNDS, AND AIDS FERTILITY.

ROAST MONKFISH WITH FENNEL, GARLIC, AND ROSEMARY

CALORIE COUNT: **118** WITH BROCCOLI **133**

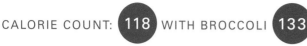

This is one ugly fish—flat head, mottled skin, those weird whiskery filaments—but monkfish has much to recommend it. Chefs love it for its firm meat that can cope with strong flavors such as the garlic, fennel, and rosemary here. Once the head has been removed, the rest of the fish is the "tail"—boneless and chunky. Discard the pink membrane, which is tough once cooked (if your fishmonger hasn't already removed it), and steep in your chosen flavors. Although monkfish was in danger in recent years, improved management has increased stocks again to sustainable levels.

A pile of steamed broccolini would be a good accompaniment.

Serves 2

10 ounces/300g monkfish
2 cloves garlic, thinly sliced
Salt and pepper
1 teaspoon olive oil
½ bulb fennel, thinly sliced
3 sprigs fresh rosemary
A generous handful of fresh curly parsley, chopped
Lemon wedges, for serving

Preheat the oven to 400°F. Slash the monkfish with a small, sharp knife and insert garlic slivers into the grooves. Season well. Lightly oil a roasting pan and place the fennel, rosemary, and fish in it, in that order. Roast uncovered for 15 to 20 minutes, till fish and fennel are cooked through. Serve with plenty of chopped parsley and lemon wedges.

NB

GARLIC IS WORTH ADDING TO ANY DISH—ITS ACTIVE INGREDIENT, ALLICIN, HELPS LOWER BLOOD PRESSURE, PROTECT CELLS, AND REDUCE FATTY DEPOSITS.[1]

GARLIC MASALA SHRIMP

CALORIE COUNT: **118**

This recipe cleverly dodges the obvious where's-the-garlic-butter question; instead, it imparts kicking flavor from the spices. There's just a bit of butter, though. When choosing warm-water shrimp, such as king and tiger, buy organic ones from a certified fishery.

Serve with plenty of wilted spinach or a salad of lemon-dressed herb leaves.

Serves 2

Masala paste

2 teaspoons cumin seeds
½ cinnamon stick, broken
3 whole cloves
1 clove garlic, minced
Salt and pepper
2 teaspoons chili powder
1 teaspoon ground turmeric
1 tablespoon vegetable oil

Shrimp

2 teaspoons butter
5 ounces/150g raw tiger shrimp, peeled and deveined
Juice of 1 lemon
A handful of fresh cilantro leaves, chopped

To make the masala paste, heat a pan. Put in the cumin, cinnamon, and cloves and toast for a minute, till fragrant. Remove from the heat and grind in a mini food processor. Add the garlic, salt and pepper, chili powder, turmeric, and oil and whiz to a paste. Add a splash of water if too thick. Melt the butter in a heavy pan, add the paste, and fry for 2 minutes. Add the shrimp and stir gently till pink, sticky, and cooked through. Top with the lemon juice and cilantro.

NB

SHRIMP DO CONTAIN CHOLESTEROL, BUT THE DIETARY TYPE DOES NOT HAVE A SIGNIFICANT IMPACT ON LEVELS OF CHOLESTEROL IN THE BLOOD.

CEVICHE WITH CILANTRO SALAD

CALORIE COUNT: 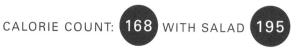 WITH SALAD

If raw fish leaves you cold, try ceviche. The acid in the citrus will "cook" the fish without heat, turning it from translucent to opalescent as you watch. This is a traditional Latin American method, and it requires, of course, the freshest fish you can muster. It works with bass, cod, and mackerel—and it is particularly good with snapper. Scallops are good, too, if very fresh and plump. Serve scallops with tarragon, dill, chives, or parsley instead of the cilantro salad.

Ceviche

5 ounces/150g very fresh red snapper fillet (or preferred fish), skinned and cut into ¾-inch cubes
Juice of 1 lime
Juice of 1 lemon
½ red onion, diced
½ teaspoon grated fresh ginger
1 red chile, seeded and finely chopped
Salt and pepper
Tabasco sauce, to taste

Salad

A handful of herby salad leaves
1 ripe tomato, chopped
A very large handful of fresh cilantro, chopped

Place all the ceviche ingredients in a nonreactive bowl. Leave to marinate till the citrus has "cooked" the fish—an hour or so. Serve with herb salad leaves, diced tomato, and cilantro.

NB

UNUSUAL FOR A WHITE LOW-FAT FISH, RED SNAPPER CONTAINS A REASONABLE AMOUNT OF VITAMIN D.

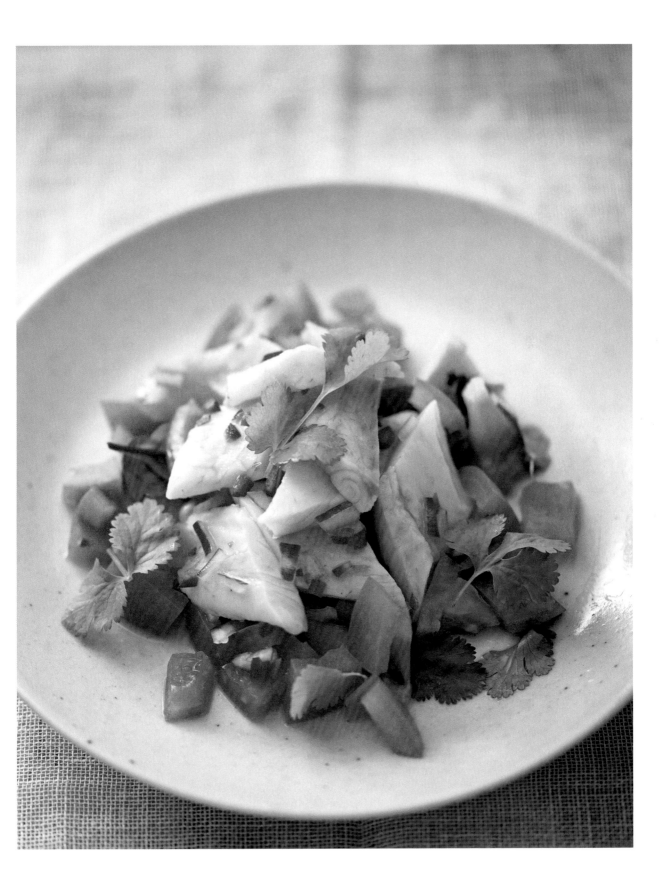

SALMON FILLET THREE MORE WAYS

CALORIE COUNT: 257

These recipes use salmon fillet (80 calories per 100g/3½ ounces) because it is easily accessible and a fish that nearly everyone likes. These recipes work equally well with other fish, too. You could push out the boat and attempt any of them with tilapia, trout, arctic char, or cod.

Broken, with Cucumber and Dill

3½ ounces/100g salmon fillet
Salt and pepper
Scant 2 ounces/50g iceberg lettuce leaves
Scant 2 ounces/50g romaine lettuce leaves
Scant 2 ounces/50g baby spinach, lamb's lettuce, or purslane
¼ seedless cucumber, quartered, cored, and sliced into crescents

Dressing

2 tablespoons unflavored low-fat yogurt
Juice of ½ lime
A handful of chopped fresh dill, plus more for garnish

Lime wedges, for garnish

Season the salmon fillet with salt and pepper and place in a bamboo steamer over boiling water. Steam till opaque. Set aside to cool. Mix the dressing. Arrange the leaves and cucumber on a plate and break the warm salmon into pieces on top. Dress and garnish with more dill and lime wedges.

NB

CUCUMBER IS ONE OF THE LOWEST-CALORIE FOODS, SO IT MAKES A GOOD FAST DAY SNACK.

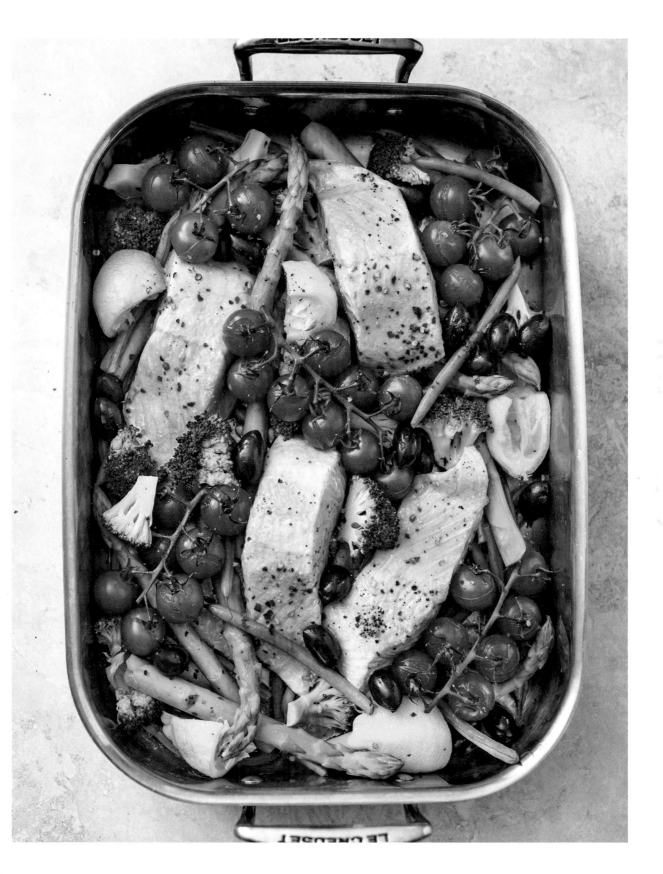

O'Kelly Fish

CALORIE COUNT: 318

Serves 4

14 ounces/400g trimmed green beans, blanched and
   refreshed
7 ounces/200g broccoli florets, blanched and refreshed
7 ounces/200g asparagus spears, trimmed, blanched, and refreshed
2 lemons
2 tablespoons olive oil
1 teaspoon red pepper flakes
Salt and pepper
A handful of black Greek olives (1 ounce/30g)
4 vines cherry tomatoes (6 to 8 tomatoes per vine), or 24 to 32 loose cherry tomatoes
Four 3½-ounce/100g salmon fillets

Preheat the oven to 400°F. Place the blanched vegetables in a large roasting pan and squeeze the juice of 1 lemon over them. Drizzle with the olive oil, season with the red pepper and salt and pepper, and mix together. Scatter in the olives and place the tomatoes on top. Lay the salmon fillets, skin side down, as a top layer, and squeeze the second lemon over the top, throwing in the rinds of both lemons. Roast for 20 minutes, or till the fish is just cooked and the vegetables are beginning to char. The tomatoes and lemon will have made a wonderful juice to spoon over the fish.

Poached, with Green Bean Salad and Tomato-Anchovy Dressing

CALORIE COUNT: **321**

Dressing

1 ripe tomato, finely chopped
1 anchovy fillet, finely chopped
1 scallion (green onion), finely chopped
1 tablespoon lemon juice
2 teaspoons olive oil

½ bulb fennel, sliced thinly
Salt and pepper
1 bay leaf
3½ ounces/100g salmon fillet
3½ ounces/100g green beans, steamed but still al dente
3½ ounces/100g sugar snap peas, lightly steamed
A handful of torn basil

Whiz the dressing ingredients in a blender or mini food processor till pureed. Set aside. Bring a pan of water to a boil; add the fennel, salt and pepper, and bay leaf; boil for 5 minutes, then remove from the heat. Add the salmon, cover, and set aside for 15 minutes. Drain the fish and break into bite-size chunks. Serve on the steamed beans and sugar snaps, along with a little fennel from the pan. Drizzle with the dressing and top with basil leaves.

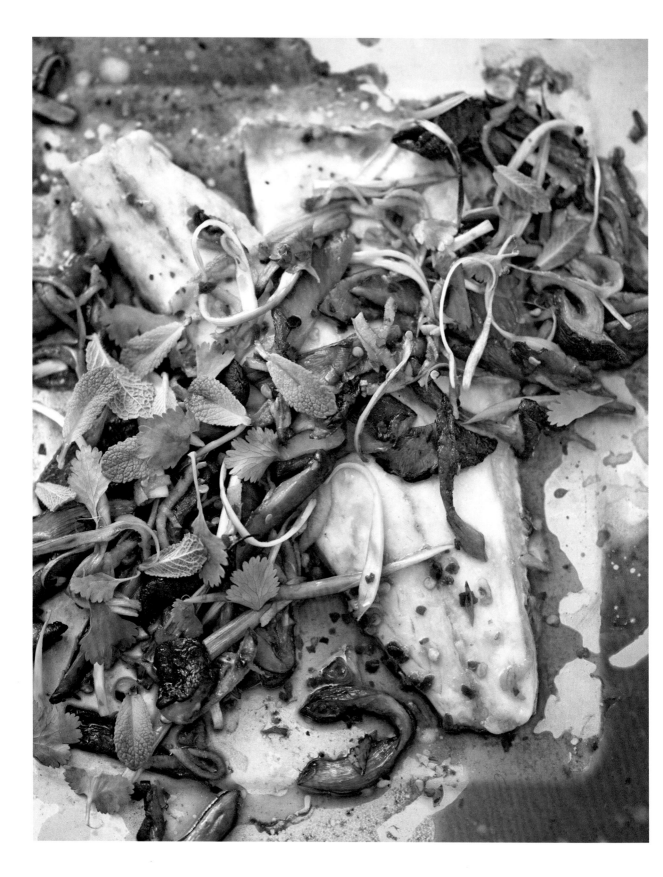

VIETNAMESE SEA BASS

CALORIE COUNT: 185

Note the delightfully minuscule calorie count. Note the fragrant aroma as it arrives on your plate, as if from heaven itself. Poetic? Well, it is.

Serves 2

2 teaspoons sesame oil
1 ounce/30g shiitake mushrooms, sliced
1 ounce/30g oyster mushrooms, sliced
Salt and pepper
1 scallion (green onion), julienned lengthwise
½ teaspoon red pepper flakes, or more to taste
½ inch/1 cm fresh ginger, thinly sliced
1 medium sea bass fillet (preferably line-caught)
1 tablespoon oyster sauce
Juice of ½ lime
1½ teaspoons soy sauce
1½ teaspoons Asian fish sauce
Fresh herb leaves, for garnish

Preheat the oven to 375°F. Heat the oil in a pan, add the mushrooms, and season. Cook till tender, 4 to 5 minutes, then combine with the scallion, red pepper, and ginger. Place the fish in a small ovenproof dish and add the mushroom mixture. Mix the oyster sauce, lime juice, soy sauce, and fish sauce. Pour over the fish, season, and bake uncovered for 10 to 15 minutes. Serve scattered with fresh herbs.

WHOLE BAKED SEA BASS WITH LEMONGRASS

CALORIE COUNT: 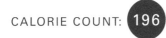 196

Delicate, aromatic, elegant, and—dare I say—so much easier than ordering out for pizza.

Serves 2

1 whole line-caught sea bass (about 1 pound/500g), gutted and cleaned
Spray oil
3 stalks lemongrass, outer leaves removed, inner stalk thinly sliced on the diagonal
1¼-inch/3 cm piece fresh ginger, peeled and julienned
2 small chiles, seeded and chopped
1 clove garlic, minced
1 teaspoon honey
Juice and zest of 1 lime
1 tablespoon olive oil
Salt and pepper

Preheat the oven to 400°F. Score the fish skin and lay on a large piece of oiled foil. Pound the lemongrass in a mortar, or grind in a mini food processor, with the ginger, chiles, garlic, honey, lime juice and zest, and olive oil. Season the fish with salt and pepper, and then rub with the lemongrass mixture inside and out, working it well into the scored skin. Wrap the foil to make a loose package and bake for 25 minutes. Let it rest for a minute before opening.

NB

LEMONGRASS CONTAINS FOLATES, MINERALS, AND ANTIOXIDANT VITAMINS—AND THAT GORGEOUS FRESH FLAVOR.

Alternatively, try this with lemon, flat-leaf parsley, and thinly sliced fennel.

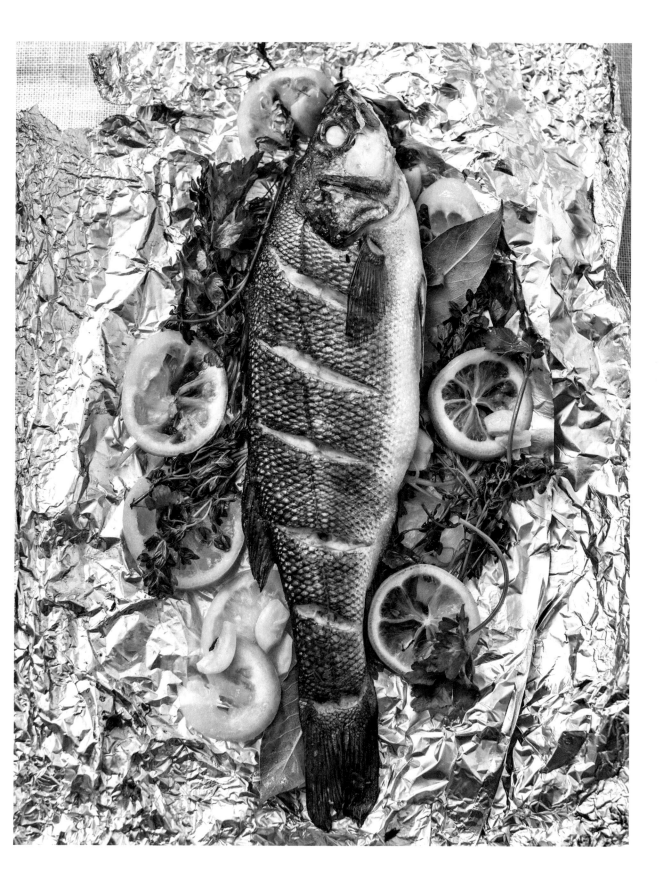

STEAMED MUSSELS IN A LIGHT TOMATO BROTH

CALORIE COUNT: 208

Fiddly food is a bit of a bonus on a fast day, and mussels are a great way to get more minerals into your diet. They remain one of the most environmentally sound fish or shellfish available. Select only those with tightly closed shells. Their plump flesh, quickly steamed in this light tomato broth, makes for an elegant little supper.

Serves 4

1 teaspoon olive oil
2 cloves garlic, finely chopped
12 ounces/350g ripe tomatoes, seeded and finely chopped
1¼ cups/300ml fish or vegetable stock
2¼ pounds/1kg farmed mussels, scrubbed, debearded if necessary
Salt and pepper
A handful of fresh parsley, chopped

Warm the oil over medium heat in a large saucepan with a tight-fitting lid. Add the garlic and cook gently for 2 minutes. Add the tomatoes and turn up the heat, cooking for a few minutes more. Add the stock and bring to a boil. Then add the mussels. Cover firmly and steam gently, shaking the pan occasionally, for 3 to 4 minutes, till the mussels have opened. Discard any that haven't. Season and serve in a deep soup bowl with the tomato broth, topped with fresh parsley.

NB

OUNCE FOR OUNCE, MUSSELS CONTAIN DOUBLE THE IRON OF RED MEAT.

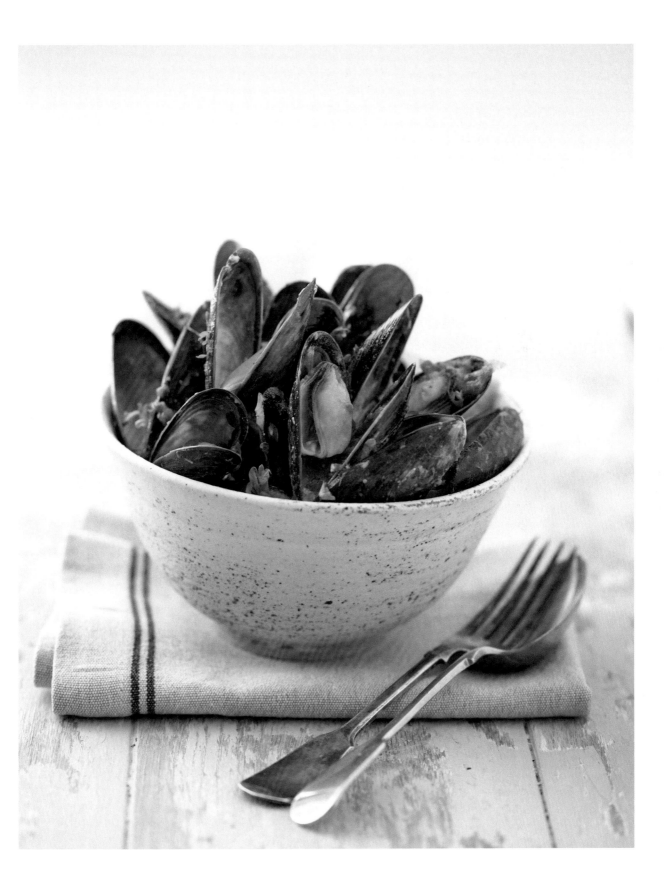

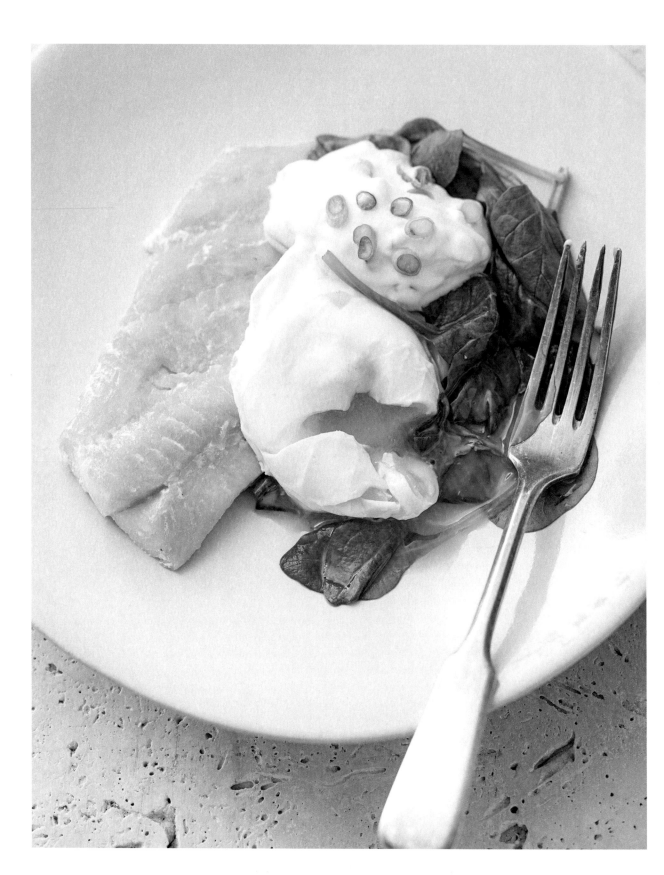

SMOKED FISH WITH SPINACH AND POACHED EGG

CALORIE COUNT: 211

There are few combinations as comforting to me as this medley—a melody, almost—of smoky haddock, dark-green spinach, and a quivering poached egg. It's a collaboration of flavors I well remember from childhood: a trad not a rad dish, but all the better for it. And the calories? Diddly-squat. You can substitute smoked trout, if you can't get smoked haddock. It's fully cooked, but you might want to heat it a bit.

3½ ounces/100g baby spinach leaves
Salt and pepper
A grating of nutmeg
3 ounces/75g undyed skinless smoked haddock fillet
1 cup/240ml 1% milk (optional)
1 medium egg
1 tablespoon Vermont Creamery crème fraîche or fromage blanc
½ scallion (green onion), finely chopped
A squeeze of lemon juice

Wilt the spinach leaves in a little salted boiling water and drain well. Stir in a pinch of nutmeg and season with black pepper. Poach the fish for 10 minutes in the milk (or microwave for 3 minutes in a covered dish). Meanwhile, poach the egg (see page 14). Serve the fish and spinach topped with egg and the crème fraîche mixed with the scallion and a squeeze of lemon.

NB

COOKED SPINACH SUPPLIES MORE ANTIOXIDANTS, SUCH AS CAROTENOIDS AND FERULIC ACID, THAN RAW.[2]

This combination of ingredients also works well baked in a ramekin. Preheat the oven to 400°F. Place a ramekin on a baking sheet. Wilt the spinach and drain well, pressing to squeeze out the moisture. Poach the fish as above till opaque, and flake with a fork. Place the spinach, flaked haddock, crème fraîche mixed with the scallion and a squeeze of lemon, and seasoning in a bowl and mix. Transfer to the ramekin, cover lightly with oiled foil, and bake for 10 to 15 minutes, then make a well in the center of the mixture and break an egg into it. Season and bake for 5 to 8 minutes more, according to how set you like your egg.

RIVER COTTAGE FISH PARCELS WITH ASIAN SPICES

CALORIE COUNT: 215

Our friend Hugh Fearnley-Whittingstall is something of a fast day fan, having lost 11 pounds in the month following Christmas. Here, then, is the kind of thing he might rustle up for a fast day supper: "Baking fish scrunched up in a foil parcel with a handful of aromatics is an easy and delicious option," says Hugh. "Fillets of gurnard, lemon sole, bream, mullet and line-caught bass all respond well to this treatment, as well as thick fillets of pollock. And it's not just fillets that benefit from the foil parcel approach. In fact, this is one of my favorite ways to cook small-to-medium fish."

Serve with wilted greens (7 ounces/200g per person), such as spinach, bok choy, or choi sum.

Serves 2

1 tablespoon peanut oil
2 bulbs fennel, trimmed, quartered, and sliced fairly thin
2 cloves garlic, thinly sliced
1 teaspoon finely chopped fresh ginger
1 small red chile, seeded and thinly sliced
2 large (5- to 7-ounce/150g to 200g) or 4 small
    (3- to 4-ounce/80g to 120g) mild white fish fillets
Salt and pepper
2 teaspoons soy sauce

Preheat the oven to 375°F. Heat half of the oil in a pan, add the fennel, and cook gently for a few minutes. Add the garlic, ginger, and chile and cook for a few minutes more, so everything starts to soften and release its flavor. Remove from heat and set aside. Take two pieces of foil, each roughly 10 inches square, and oil well with the remaining oil. Pile the fennel mixture in the middle of each one. Season the fish fillets generously and curl around the fennel mixture—either 2 small fillets or 1 large per parcel. Sprinkle a little soy sauce and black pepper over each pile, then bring up the sides of the foil and scrunch together tightly to form well-sealed but baggy parcels. Place in a baking pan, and bake for 15 minutes. Open up the steaming, fragrant parcels and pile the contents, including all the lovely juices, onto warm plates.

NB

STEAMING "EN PAPILLOTE" SEALS IN FLAVOR AND REQUIRES VERY LITTLE ADDED FAT.

LEEK AND LEMON SHRIMP

CALORIE COUNT: 225

A favorite quick supper at my sister-in-law Clara's house—one of those eat-from-the-bowl winners that take the sweat out of cooking.

Serves 2

2 leeks, washed and sliced into 1¼-inch chunks
¾-inch piece fresh ginger, peeled and grated
¼ red chile, seeded
1 clove garlic, minced
Juice of 1 lemon
1½ teaspoons olive oil
3½ ounces/100g shrimp, precooked or raw, peeled and deveined
Salt and pepper
A large handful of fresh cilantro, chopped

Place the leeks in a steamer and cook for 4 to 5 minutes, till tender. Combine the ginger, chile, garlic, and lemon juice in a mini food processor (or chop finely by hand). Sauté the paste in the olive oil for a couple of minutes before adding the shrimp. Cook till the shrimp are fully heated or done to your liking. Add the leeks and mix through. Season, sprinkle with cilantro, and serve.

NB

LEEKS ARE LOW IN CALORIES (22 PER 3½ OUNCES) AND LOW-GI, TOO.

SKEWERED MONKFISH WITH
BALSAMIC COLESLAW

CALORIE COUNT: 226

These chunky fish skewers will work well on a barbecue, too (give them a little spray with oil before they go on the grill to stop them from sticking). The lime will swell, buckle, and burst in the heat, while the crisp chile-balsamic coleslaw makes for the perfect partnership. Works with shrimp too, of course.

5 ounces/150g monkfish, cut into thick chunks
1 tablespoon lime juice
Salt and pepper
1 clove garlic, minced
Lime wedges
Kaffir lime leaves (omit if you can't find fresh ones)
Spray oil
1 or 2 wooden skewers

Coleslaw

Scant 2 ounces/50g snow peas, blanched and refreshed, halved crosswise
Scant 2 ounces/50g sugar snap peas, blanched and refreshed, halved crosswise
Scant 2 ounces/50g Chinese cabbage, sliced
1 scallion (green onion), thinly sliced lengthwise

Dressing

1 tablespoon soy sauce
1½ teaspoons balsamic vinegar
1 teaspoon lime juice
1½ teaspoons sesame oil
1 teaspoon red pepper flakes

Spray oil
1 tablespoon toasted sesame seeds, for garnish

Marinate the fish in the lime juice, salt, pepper, and garlic and allow to rest while you prepare the slaw and dressing. Combine the snow peas and sugar snap peas with the sliced cabbage and scallion. For the dressing, whisk the ingredients in a small bowl. Skewer the monkfish pieces, alternating fish with a lime wedge and a lime leaf. Heat a

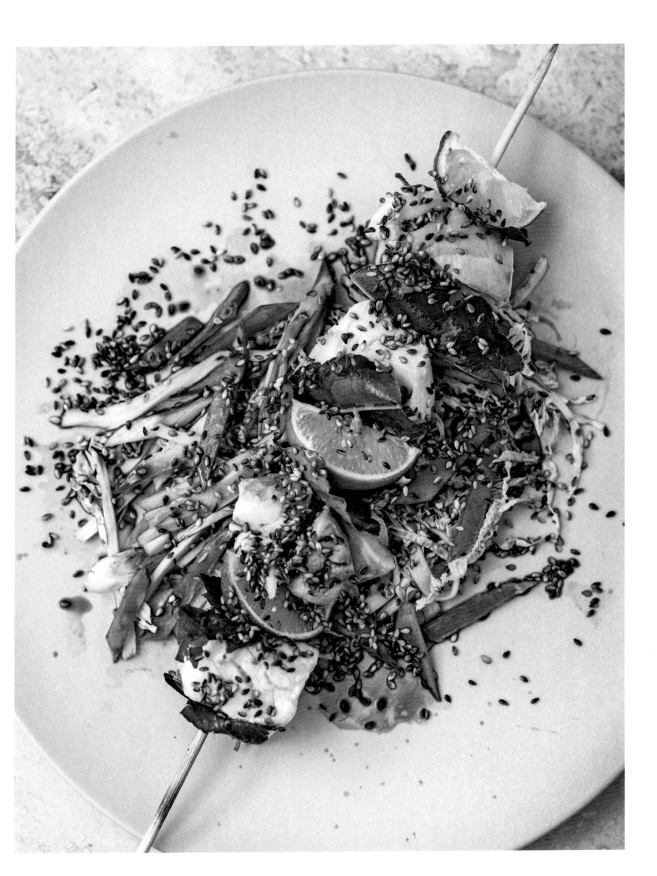

skillet till hot, spray with oil, and cook the skewers for 2 minutes on each of the 4 sides. Dress the slaw, garnish with sesame seeds, and top with fish skewers.

NB

EATING CRUCIFEROUS VEGETABLES—INCLUDING ALL KINDS OF CABBAGE—CAN HELP GUARD AGAINST CANCER.[3]

STIR-FRY LEMONGRASS SHRIMP WITH SHIRATAKI NOODLES

CALORIE COUNT: 230

Committed FastDieters will already know all about shirataki noodles. Made from a water-soluble fiber, they boast no carbs, have virtually no calories, and take no time at all to prepare. That said, they taste of nothing in particular, so here lemongrass and ginger do their mighty work.

1½ teaspoons sesame oil
½ clove garlic, minced
½ stalk lemongrass, outer leaves removed, inner stalk finely chopped
½ red chile, finely chopped
1 teaspoon grated fresh ginger
1 Kaffir lime leaf, shredded
6 tiger shrimp, raw and shell on
1½ teaspoons Asian fish sauce
1 tablespoon soy sauce
2 teaspoons lime juice
1 ounce/30g bean sprouts
3½ ounces/100g shirataki noodles
Fresh cilantro leaves and lime wedges, for garnish
1 tablespoon/10g unsalted peanuts, chopped

Heat the sesame oil in a pan and cook the garlic, lemongrass, chile, and ginger till soft. Add the lime leaf and 3 tablespoons water. Simmer for 5 minutes. Add the shrimp, fish sauce, soy sauce, lime juice, and bean sprouts. Cook till the shrimp are pink. Rinse the noodles in warm water as instructed and add to the shrimp. Serve with cilantro, lime wedges, and peanuts.

NB

SHIRATAKI NOODLES ARE MADE FROM FATLESS WATER-SOLUBLE FIBER: GLUTEN-FREE, ZERO CARBS, ZERO CALORIES.

ALLEGRA McEVEDY'S SCALLOPS WITH ASPARAGUS

CALORIE COUNT: 256

Allegra is a brilliant cook and a dear friend. She says: "At the height of the season, I try to have asparagus at least three times a week, and it still feels like a treat every time . . . The dark green leaves of the garlic plant come into season about the same time as asparagus. Use baby spinach if there are no garlic leaves, but do try to hunt them down as they are a whole new kind of fabulous."

Serves 6

Scant ½ cup/100ml extra virgin olive oil
2 cloves garlic
1 tablespoon chopped fresh mint
1 tablespoon chopped fresh dill
1 tablespoon chopped fresh basil
1 tablespoon chopped fresh chervil
A squeeze of lemon juice
Salt and pepper
2 bunches asparagus (allow 3 to 6 spears per serving)
12 to 18 sea scallops (2 or 3 per person, depending on size), muscle tab removed
5 ounces/150g garlic or ramp leaves, cut into 1¼-inch lengths, or baby spinach

Heat the olive oil and garlic very gently for 5 to 7 minutes. Let cool to room temperature, then discard the garlic. Once completely cool (otherwise the herbs will discolor), stir in the chopped herbs, a squeeze of lemon, and some seasoning. Slice the asparagus on the diagonal into 1- to 1½-inch pieces and set aside.

Preheat the broiler. Line a broiler pan with foil, insert the slotted top, and heat on the highest shelf under the broiler. Pat the scallops dry and season well. Place the scallops (not touching) on the broiler pan and broil for 2 to 4 minutes on each side, depending on size, till opaque with a small amount of resistance when you squeeze them.

Meanwhile, steam the asparagus for 2 minutes, covered, in about ¾ cup/150ml water in a large skillet. Uncover, add the garlic leaves, and cook to let the water evaporate. Add two-thirds of the herb dressing to the vegetables and toss well. Divide among six plates and top with the scallops. Drizzle generously with the remaining dressing.

NB

ACCORDING TO PRELIMINARY STUDIES, ASPARAGUS CONTAINS SUBSTANCES THAT MAY HELP TO ALLEVIATE HANGOVERS.[4]

WHITE FISH STEW WITH ORANGE AND FENNEL

CALORIE COUNT: 268

Greek legend has it that a fennel stalk carried the coal that passed down knowledge from the gods to men. I couldn't possibly say, but I do know that this marriage of fennel, firm fish, and zingy orange verges on the divine.

Use clean trim and bones from only nonoily fish to make stock. Save shrimp shells, and when buying filleted fish, ask for the bones; freeze them for later use. Any extra stock can be frozen.

Serves 4

Fish stock

1¼ pounds/500g fish bones and trim and shrimp shells
1 onion, quartered
1 stalk celery
Fennel trimmings (see stew ingredients below)
1 tablespoon peppercorns

Stew

2 tablespoons olive oil
1 onion, thinly sliced
3 cloves garlic, thinly sliced
1 small bulb fennel, trimmed and thinly sliced
1 teaspoon coriander seeds
1 cup/250ml fish stock
Juice of 1 orange and 2 strips of peel
One 14-ounce/400g can diced tomatoes
2 bay leaves
½ teaspoon dried herbes de Provence or dried tarragon
A pinch of saffron threads
Salt and pepper
1 pound 7 ounces/750g white fish fillets (such as pollock, monkfish, or halibut),
    in large chunks
8 tiger shrimp, shell on (preferably with heads)
A large handful of fresh parsley, chopped

To make your own stock, combine the ingredients in a deep saucepan and cover with water. Bring to a boil, then skim off any froth. Lower the heat and simmer for about

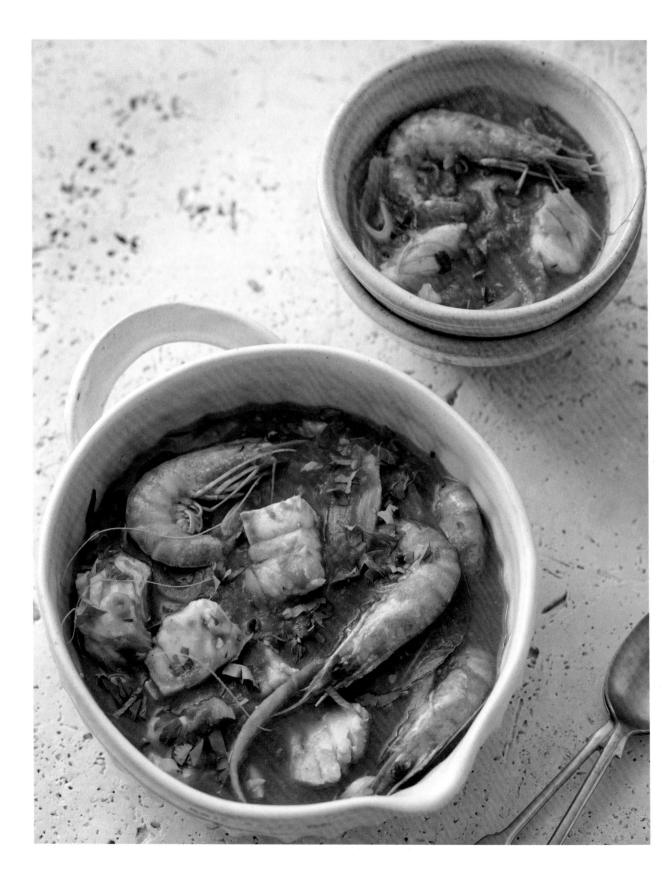

45 minutes. Strain the stock and discard the solids. Refrigerate or freeze what you don't need for the stew.

Heat the oil in a large nonstick saucepan and gently sauté the onion, garlic, fennel, and coriander for 15 minutes, till tender. Add the stock, orange juice and peel, tomatoes, 1¾ cups cold water, bay leaves, herbs, and saffron. Season and simmer for 20 to 25 minutes. Add the fish, then the shrimp. Cover and cook for about 4 minutes more, till the fish and shrimp are cooked through. Serve piping hot and scattered with fresh parsley.

NB

A GOOD STOCK IS THE BACKBONE HERE—FULL OF MINERALS, FULL OF FLAVOR.

SEARED SESAME TUNA FOUR WAYS

CALORIE COUNT: 317

This uses tuna loin, which ought to be eaten rare. That way, it melts in the mouth and is a real treat to eat. Tuna is rich in oils and provides a great source of lean protein, but buy it and eat it with care.

7 ounces/200g fresh tuna loin
Olive oil
Salt and pepper
2 teaspoons sesame seeds

Heat a cast-iron skillet till very hot. Rub the tuna with a little olive oil and season well. Roll in the sesame seeds. Cook on each side for 30 seconds, leaving the interior as rare as you dare. Serve sliced with one of the following.

NB

ONLY FRESH TUNA COUNTS TOWARD OILY FISH INTAKE; CANNED TUNA LOSES MOST OF ITS OMEGA-3 FATS DURING THE CANNING PROCESS.

Soy-Mirin Dressing

CALORIE COUNT: ADD 19

Make a dressing from 1 tablespoon mirin, 1 tablespoon soy sauce, and 1 tablespoon rice vinegar. Top the tuna with scant 2 ounces/50g shredded daikon radish, scant 2 ounces/50g julienned seedless cucumber, and a handful each of fresh mint leaves and cilantro. Drizzle with the dressing.

Lemongrass Dipping Sauce

CALORIE COUNT: ADD 28

Combine 1 tablespoon Asian fish sauce; 1 tablespoon lime juice; ½ teaspoon brown sugar; ½ stalk lemongrass, finely chopped; ½ red chile, sliced; and ½ clove garlic, chopped. Spoon over the tuna. This dip works well with other fish, too. Try it with shrimp, lemon sole, or flounder. Sole has a low oil content, so cook it quickly to avoid drying it out.

Chile Green Beans

CALORIE COUNT: ADD 50

Heat a little sesame oil and sauté 1 chopped shallot, 1 teaspoon nigella or fennel seeds, and ½ teaspoon red pepper flakes. Add a handful of blanched thin green beans (scant 2 ounces) and ½ tablespoon oyster sauce. Cook till the beans are tender.

Salsa Verde

CALORIE COUNT: ADD 121

Make enough salsa for 4 servings (it will keep in the fridge for 4 to 5 days) from 1 teaspoon Dijon mustard, 3 tablespoons/50ml extra virgin olive oil, and the juice and grated zest of ½ lemon. Whisk or shake to emulsify. Add 2 finely chopped anchovy fillets; a handful each of fresh flat-leaf parsley, mint, basil, and tarragon leaves, all chopped; and 1 teaspoon chopped rinsed capers. Crush a garlic clove to a paste with salt and add. Mix well, and drizzle over the tuna.

ALLEGRA McEVEDY'S BAKE-IN-THE-BAG FISH WITH PRESERVED LEMON COUSCOUS

CALORIE COUNT: 364

Says my friend Allegra: "This is just about the healthiest and easiest supper I know. It's an all-in-one, steam-in-the-bag number, which lets the flavors just hang out and party together without getting busted. The real joy of this is what happens to the couscous, which cooks in the fish juices and greedily absorbs all the aromatics. If you can't get monkfish, any fresh, white fish will do. The bags can be made up a few hours ahead of time and kept in the fridge."

Serves 6

9 ounces/250g instant couscous
2 teaspoons ground cumin
1 teaspoon cumin seeds
6 scallions (green onions), thinly sliced
2 preserved lemons, rinds only, coarsely chopped
2 teaspoons/10g coarsely chopped fresh cilantro
18 cherry tomatoes, quartered
Salt and pepper
About 1¾ cups water
1 teaspoon saffron threads
3 tablespoons olive oil
Spray oil
2 small bulbs fennel, halved, cored, and sliced
2½ pounds/1.2kg thick fish fillets (such as monkfish, halibut, or turbot), cut into 6 portions

Preheat the oven to 400°F. Combine the couscous, ground and whole cumin, scallions, preserved lemons, cilantro, and tomatoes in a bowl. Season. Bring ¾ cup water to a boil; remove from the heat and add the saffron. Let steep for a minute or so. Stir the olive oil and saffron water into the couscous. Take six pieces of foil, each roughly 10 inches square, and spray lightly with oil. Divide the fennel among the sheets. Top with the couscous mixture and the fish. Fold the foil together and crimp tightly on two sides, leaving the top open. Pour 3 tablespoons water into each bag. Seal and place in a baking pan. Bake for 15 to 20 minutes, till the bags are nicely puffed up. Present the bags to your guests (on plates) to eat straight out of the foil—very little washing up!

NB

STEAMING HELPS PRESERVE WATER-SOLUBLE VITAMINS THAT CAN ORDINARILY GET LOST IN BOILING.

TUNA FAGIOLI

CALORIE COUNT:

This is one of the quick and tasty Italian dishes I grew up on, and today it makes the perfect fast day supper—comfortably low in all the things you ought to avoid, but sky-high in flavor. It is simplicity itself to prepare, a real cupboard standby, and—like chili con carne—it tastes even better the following day. You could drain the tuna to save on calories, though you'd need to replace it with olive oil if you do; some oil is essential here. But don't panic. Not much.

Serves 2

One 3-ounce can white tuna in oil or half a 6-ounce can, undrained
One 14-ounce/400g can great northern, white kidney, cannellini, or butter beans,
    or chickpeas, drained
½ red onion, thinly sliced or chopped
1 tablespoon white wine vinegar
Juice of ½ lemon
1 clove garlic, minced
2 large ripe tomatoes, sliced
A handful of fresh flat-leaf parsley leaves
Coarse sea salt and pepper

Put the tuna, beans, onion, vinegar, lemon juice, and garlic in a bowl. Mix and leave to settle for 30 minutes. Serve with sliced tomatoes generously sprinkled with parsley and coarse sea salt and pepper.

NB

THE BENEFICIAL SULFUR COMPOUNDS IN ONIONS CAN BE DESTROYED IN COOKING; HERE, RAW RED ONION IS LESS AGGRESSIVE THAN WHITE.

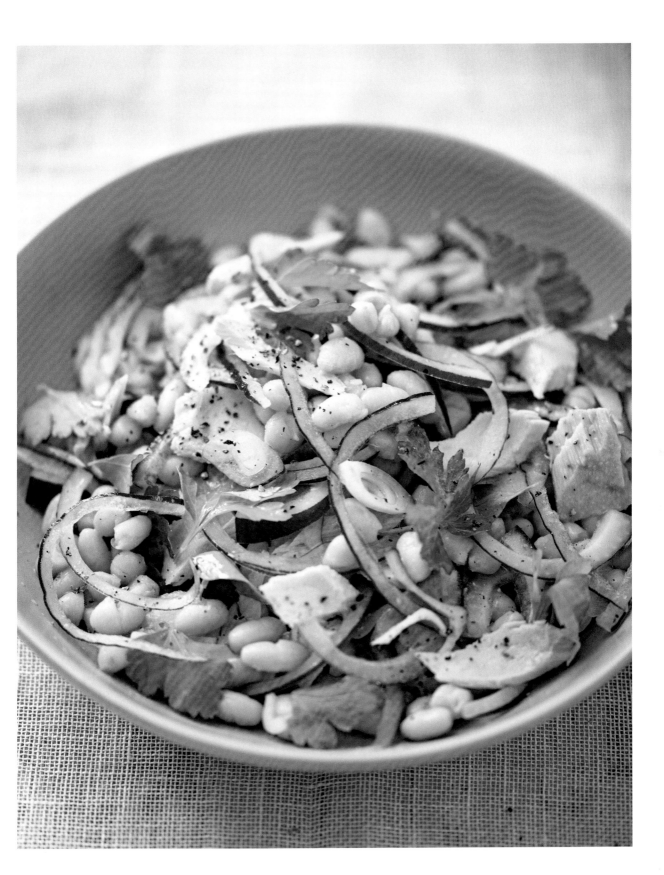

HERRING WITH A SPICED ALMOND CRUST

CALORIE COUNT: 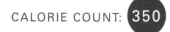 350

Ah, the underrated, overlooked herring. They fill our waters and are modest, inexpensive, and a fine way to get your omega-3 fix.

2 herring fillets (about 3½ ounces/100g)
Scant 1 ounce/25g whole blanched almonds
A handful of fresh flat-leaf parsley, chopped
½ teaspoon grated orange zest
1 clove garlic, minced
½ teaspoon ground cumin
A pinch of red pepper flakes
Juice of ½ lemon
Salt and pepper
Lemon wedges, for serving

Preheat the oven to 350°F. Wash the herring, dry, and set to one side. Combine the almonds, parsley, orange zest, garlic, cumin, red pepper flakes, and lemon juice in a mini food processor and pulse to a paste. Season. Rub the fish with the paste and place in a small shallow roasting pan. Bake for 8 to 10 minutes, till the fish is cooked through. Serve with plenty of lemon.

NB

HERRING PROVIDES HIGH-QUALITY PROTEIN AND GOOD FATS FOR LITTLE COST.

CALORIE COUNT: 240

Or rub with 1 tablespoon store-bought tapenade instead of the almond paste.

CALORIE COUNT: 246

Or coat with the juice of 1 lime, roll in 2 teaspoons all-purpose flour, and season with plenty of cracked black pepper and salt.

CALORIE COUNT: 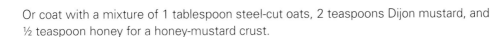 289

Or coat with a mixture of 1 tablespoon steel-cut oats, 2 teaspoons Dijon mustard, and ½ teaspoon honey for a honey-mustard crust.

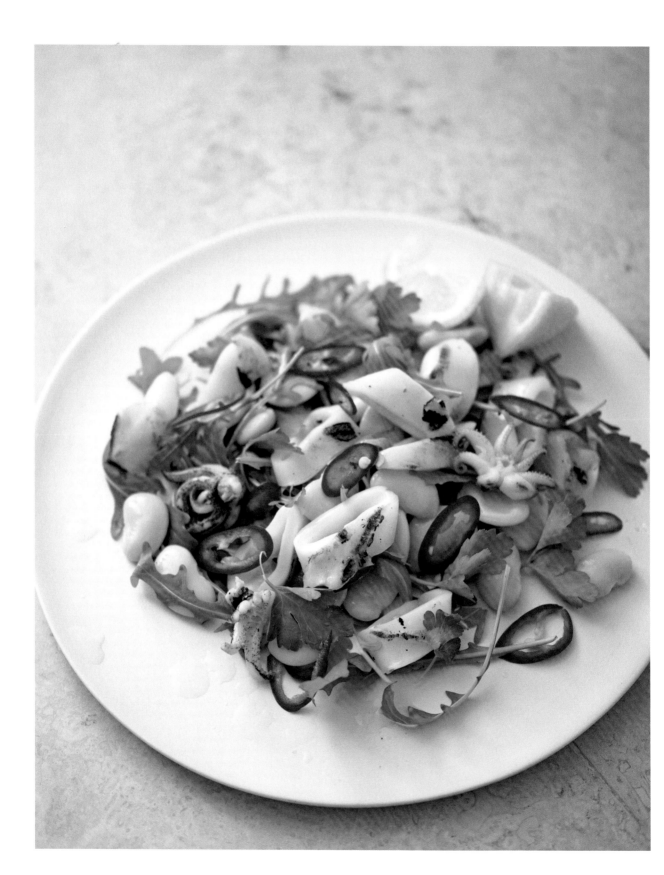

CHARRED SQUID WITH LIMA BEANS AND CHILE

CALORIE COUNT: 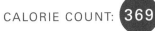 369

A glorious collision of flavor and texture, and marvelously on-message for a fast day supper. It's not dirt-cheap in calories, but what can we say? You get what you pay for.

7 ounces/200g squid, cleaned and trimmed
Salt and pepper
7 ounces/200g butter beans, drained
1 tablespoon chopped fresh parsley, plus more for serving
1½ teaspoons lemon juice
A generous handful of baby arugula
1 teaspoon olive oil
1 red chile, thinly sliced
A squeeze of lime

Score the squid and season. Gently heat the beans, adding the parsley and a little of the lemon juice. Heat a cast-iron grill pan till almost smoking. Cook the squid for a minute on each side, till slightly blackened here and there. Dress the arugula with the remaining lemon juice, the olive oil, salt and pepper, and the chile. Slice the squid and mix into the leaves. Serve with a squeeze of lime, more parsley, and the seasoned beans.

NB

SQUID IS LOW IN SATURATED FATS. JUST DON'T BATTER AND FRY IT ON A FAST DAY . . .

ROASTED SARDINES WITH MOROCCAN SPICES

CALORIE COUNT: **399**

If you want to combine all your concerns—physiological, financial, environmental—in one fine little fish, look to sardines: loaded with protein, high in omega 3s, cheap cheap cheap, and impressively light in contaminants, since they live low on the food chain. Go for sardines caught in traditional drift or ring nets, and be generous with the parsley.

1½ teaspoons cumin seeds
1½ teaspoons coriander seeds
2 cloves garlic, chopped
A handful of fresh cilantro, plus more for serving
A handful of fresh flat-leaf parsley
Cayenne pepper, to taste
1½ teaspoons paprika
Juice of ½ lemon
2 teaspoons flaxseed oil
2 large sardines, cleaned, gutted, and filleted (about 7 ounces/200g)
Lemon wedges and thinly sliced red onion, for serving

Toast the cumin and coriander seeds in a dry skillet, then grind to a powder in a mini food processor. (If in a hurry, you could use 1 tablespoon garam masala instead.) Add the garlic, herbs, cayenne, paprika, and lemon juice and pulse to chop. Emulsify with the flaxseed oil. Slash the sardine skins and rub with the mixture. Leave to rest for 2 hours in the fridge. Roast for 8 to 10 minutes at 400°F. Serve with fresh lemon wedges, more cilantro, and a scatter of thinly sliced red onion.

NB

A DIET RICH IN OMEGA-3 FATTY ACIDS—SARDINES ARE A BRILLIANT SOURCE—HELPS TO CUT YOUR RISK OF HEART DISEASE AND SOME CANCERS.[5]

SEARED MACKEREL ON A RAINBOW SALAD

CALORIE COUNT: 457

In the United States, mackerel ticks all the boxes: great taste, full of beneficent oils, relatively cheap . . . and through careful fisheries management, it is considered the most sustainable.

One 3½-ounce/100g mackerel fillet
Salt and pepper
Spray oil
½ yellow bell pepper and ½ red bell pepper, thinly sliced
½ red onion, thinly sliced
1 medium carrot, peeled and shredded

Dressing

1½ teaspoons crunchy peanut butter
3 tablespoons lime juice
1 teaspoon Asian fish sauce
1 clove garlic, minced
¾-inch piece fresh ginger, peeled and grated
1 stalk lemongrass, outer leaves removed, inner stalk finely chopped or minced
1 teaspoon agave nectar
Chopped red chile, to taste
Lemon wedges and fresh cilantro leaves, for serving

Score the mackerel fillet and season well. Spray lightly with oil and sear in a hot skillet till the skin is crisp. Mix the bell peppers, onion, and carrot and place on a plate. Combine the dressing ingredients. Place the warm fish on the vegetable salad and serve drizzled with 1 tablespoon dressing and plenty of lemon wedges and fresh cilantro leaves.

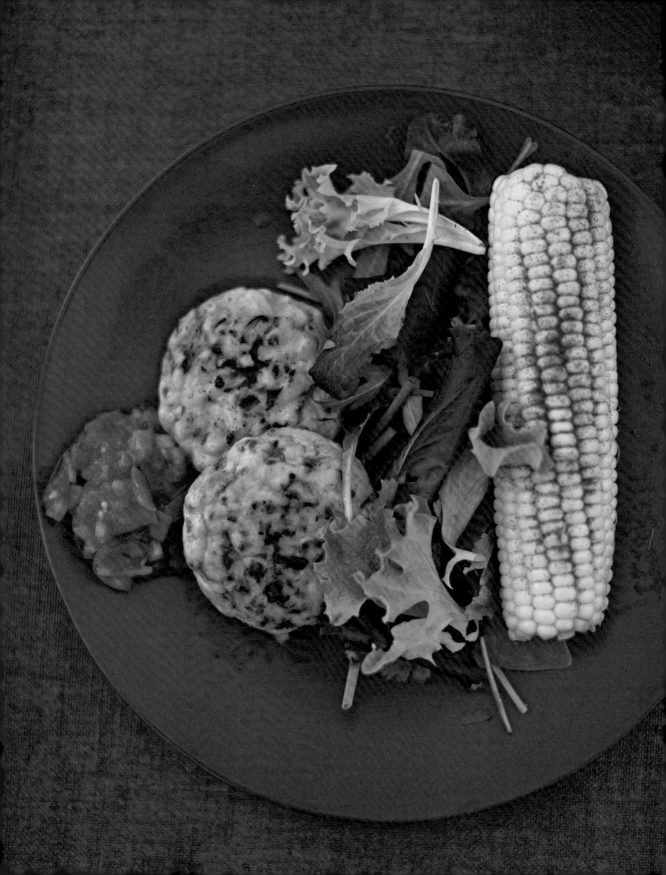

CHAPTER NINE

meat & poultry

CUMIN-SCENTED TURKEY BURGERS WITH TOMATO SALSA

CALORIE COUNT: **174** OR WITH CORN ON THE COB, LEAVES,

AND 1 TABLESPOON SALSA **333**

Swapping out beef for turkey will slash the calories in a burger (and, incidentally, the cost). But you do need a little egg to bind it all together in a steady embrace, otherwise the meat is liable to dry out and collapse before your very eyes.

4½ ounces/125g ground turkey
1 scallion (green onion), finely chopped
1 small egg, beaten
½ red chile, finely chopped
1 clove garlic, minced
½ teaspoon ground cumin
½ teaspoon ground coriander
Salt and pepper
Herby salad leaves, Classic Tomato Salsa (page 206), and
    1 ear corn (boiled and dusted with paprika), for serving

Combine the turkey, scallion, 1 tablespoon of the egg, the chile, garlic, cumin, and coriander. Season with salt and pepper. Leave to marinate for half an hour in the fridge. Shape into 2 patties and broil or grill for 5 to 7 minutes on each side, till cooked through. Serve with dressed herby salad leaves, Classic Tomato Salsa, and corn on the cob.

BAKED PORK TENDERLOIN WITH FENNEL

CALORIE COUNT: 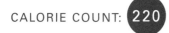 220

Fennel and pork are the best of friends, and they probably converse in Italian. This is a flavorful, lip-smacking dish, full of good things for relatively little calorie cost.

Serves 2

2 teaspoons fennel seeds, lightly crushed
Coarse sea salt and cracked black pepper
1 pork tenderloin, about 10 ounces/300g
Spray oil
⅔ cup/200ml chicken stock
2 cloves garlic, minced
2 medium bulbs fennel, trimmed (keep the fronds for garnish) and quartered
½ teaspoon olive oil
A good squeeze of lemon juice
Lemon wedges, for serving

Preheat the oven to 350°F. Sprinkle the crushed fennel seeds and plenty of salt and pepper onto a piece of parchment paper. Spray the tenderloin with a little oil, then roll in the seasonings. Sear in a hot pan for a minute on each side to seal and color the meat. Remove the pork from the pan, lower the heat, and add the stock and minced garlic to deglaze the pan. Cook for 2 minutes till heated through and the garlic begins to soften. Place the fennel in a small baking pan; add the garlicky stock, olive oil, and lemon juice; season, and place the pork on top. Bake for 15 to 20 minutes, covering loosely with foil if necessary to keep the meat moist.

Remove the pork from the oven and let it rest on a cutting board, returning the fennel to the oven for 5 minutes more to further reduce remaining liquid. Slice the pork into thick medallions and serve on a bed of fennel, drizzled with pan juices and decorated with fennel fronds and a lemon wedge or two.

GREEN PAPAYA SALAD WITH CHARGRILLED BEEF

CALORIE COUNT: 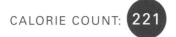 221

Unripe or green papaya is the foundation for this sparky *som tam* salad, bristling with Thai taste and chile heat. Christopher Columbus called the papaya "the fruit of the angels." A shredded green one might well be the perfect raw food. The salad is oil-free, too. Bingo.

This combination of ingredients also works well with grilled shrimp.

Dressing

1 clove garlic, minced
½ red chile, finely chopped
1 teaspoon palm sugar or light brown sugar
1 tablespoon Asian fish sauce
1 tablespoon lime juice

Salad and garnish

½ green papaya, peeled and finely shredded or julienned
¼ large seedless cucumber, cored and julienned
1 scallion (green onion), sliced
A handful of mixed fresh Thai basil, mint, and cilantro leaves

3½ ounces/100g sirloin steak
Lime wedges, for serving
Pomegranate seeds (optional)

Place the garlic, chile, sugar, fish sauce, and lime juice in a bowl and stir. Add the salad ingredients, and toss to dress. Grill the steak to your liking—it's best if pink—and let rest. Slice and serve with lime wedges on top of the dressed salad. You could add a scatter of pomegranate seeds.

NB

HALF A PAPAYA PROVIDES 50 PERCENT YOUR RECOMMENDED DAILY AMOUNT OF VITAMIN C.

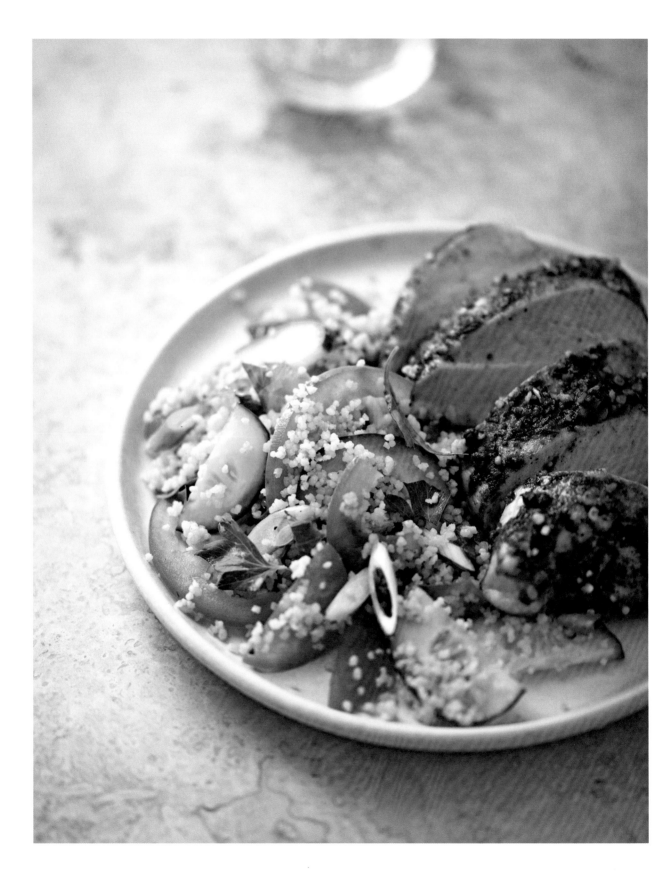

CHICKEN BREAST EIGHT WAYS

CALORIE COUNT: 195

Yes, I know. Chicken is a bore. You're not supposed to order it in restaurants—everyone will yawn and the chef will mark you down as a wuss for not ordering his fricasseed sweetbreads. But. Most of us love it and we certainly eat a lot of the stuff. Chicken fillets are simple to prepare, low in calories (about 127 per fillet), quick to cook—and when teamed with powerhouse flavors like these, you can't get a much better weekday supper, especially if you buy a fine free-range, organic bird. Be sure to remove the skin to lessen the calorie load, though if you are going to roast a chicken breast, keep the skin on till after cooking to prevent the meat from drying out (the inarguable scourge of chicken dinners everywhere).

Lime Chicken Salad, Szechuan Style

A firm favorite in our house—tangy, easy, and somehow sumptuous without being calorific. It plays on some of the classic ingredients of Thai cooking (fish sauce, lime, cilantro), a reliable foundation for fantastic fast day flavor.

Olive oil
1 skin-on, boneless 4-ounce/110g chicken breast
Salt and pepper
½ medium seedless cucumber, halved lengthwise, cored, and
    cut on the diagonal into crescents
A handful of fresh cilantro, including stems, finely chopped
A handful of fresh mint leaves
½ teaspoon Szechuan peppercorns, crushed
1 tablespoon Asian fish sauce
1 teaspoon sesame oil
1 scallion (green onion), thinly sliced on the diagonal
2 tablespoons lime juice
3 ounces/80g shredded iceberg lettuce
Lime wedges, for serving

Preheat the oven to 375°F. Oil the chicken breast lightly before seasoning with salt and pepper. Bake, covered, till cooked through and the juices run clear, about 20 minutes. Allow to cool. Remove the skin and tear the chicken into shreds. Place in a bowl with the cucumber and most of the cilantro and mint. Make a dressing with the Szechuan pepper, fish sauce, sesame oil, scallion, and lime juice, and season with salt and pepper. Combine with the chicken and serve on the lettuce, garnished with lime wedges and the remaining cilantro and mint.

Masala Style with Raita

CALORIE COUNT: **199** WITH SPINACH **219**

Marinate a skinless, boneless chicken breast in the juice of ½ lemon; ½ clove garlic, minced; ½ teaspoon ground cumin; 1 crushed cardamom pod; a large pinch of ground cloves; ½ teaspoon ground fenugreek; ½ teaspoon ground turmeric; a pinch of cayenne pepper; salt and pepper; and 1 teaspoon grated fresh ginger. Add a squeeze of lime. Refrigerate for at least an hour, or as long as overnight. Grill or broil the chicken for 7 minutes on each side and serve with 2 tablespoons unflavored low-fat yogurt combined with chopped cucumber, mint, and a sprinkle of cumin seeds (or see raita recipe on page 208). This also goes with 3½ ounces/100g wilted spinach.

Teriyaki with Sesame Seeds

CALORIE COUNT: **227**

Mix 1 tablespoon soy sauce, 1 tablespoon sake, 2 tablespoons mirin, 3 tablespoons water, 1 teaspoon grated fresh ginger, and ½ teaspoon sugar. Heat and gently simmer a skinless, boneless chicken breast in the broth till cooked through, 15 to 20 minutes. Remove the chicken from the broth and allow to rest under foil. Bring the broth back to a boil and reduce to make a sauce, stirring occasionally, till glossy and slightly sticky, about 5 minutes. Dry-toast 1 tablespoon sesame seeds till golden brown. Slice the chicken and serve with the sauce, sprinkled with the sesame seeds, and a good quantity of steamed bok choy.

Summer Poached with Lean Greens

CALORIE COUNT: 252

Bring a pan of water to a boil and add a handful of chopped cilantro stems, 3 peppercorns, 1 teaspoon grated ginger, 1 coarsely chopped shallot, and 1 teaspoon coarse sea salt. Add a skinless, boneless chicken breast and simmer for 15 to 20 minutes till cooked through. Blanch scant 2 ounces/50g broccoli florets, scant 2 ounces/50g sugar snap peas, scant 2 ounces/50g asparagus spears, and 3 ounces/75g baby spinach leaves for a minute in a separate pan of boiling water; drain, refresh, and dry on paper towels. Remove the chicken from the broth and slice. Serve on top of the vegetables, and drizzle with a dressing made from ½ teaspoon red pepper flakes, 1 teaspoon raw agave nectar, 1½ teaspoons rice vinegar, 1 tablespoon lime juice, 1 tablespoon Asian fish sauce, a pinch of ground star anise, ½ teaspoon garlic powder, salt, and pepper. Garnish with cilantro and mint leaves and lime wedges.

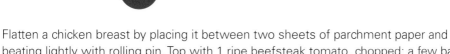

Skewered Italian

CALORIE COUNT: 260

Flatten a chicken breast by placing it between two sheets of parchment paper and beating lightly with rolling pin. Top with 1 ripe beefsteak tomato, chopped; a few basil leaves; and 2 teaspoons freshly grated Parmesan cheese. Season, roll up, skewer with a toothpick, and broil under medium heat, turning once, till done. Serve with a large helping of broccolini or some grilled zucchini strips.

French Tarragon and Lemon

CALORIE COUNT: 267

Cut a skinless, boneless chicken breast into strips and sauté in 1 teaspoon olive oil till golden, 5 to 6 minutes, moving the pieces around to prevent sticking (add a little water if they do stick). Remove from the heat and add 1 tablespoon crème fraîche or fromage blanc, the juice of ½ lemon, and a generous tablespoon of chopped fresh tarragon. Season and serve with scant 2 ounces/50g each of steamed snow peas and sugar snap peas. Garnish with tarragon sprigs.

Romano Peppers and Spinach

CALORIE COUNT: 290

Lightly steam a skinless, boneless chicken breast till cooked through, 15 minutes. Heat 1 teaspoon olive oil in a pan. Slice an orange bell pepper and a red bell pepper and add to the pan, together with a sprig of rosemary, the juice of ½ lemon, and 1 sliced garlic clove, and sauté for 3 minutes more. Add scant ½ cup/100ml water and allow to reduce and become sticky. Add a handful of spinach leaves for the final 2 minutes of cooking, and serve with the sliced steamed chicken breast, a few salt flakes, and a grating of fresh lemon zest.

Harissa-Spiked

CALORIE COUNT: 300

Smear a skinless, boneless chicken breast with 2 teaspoons harissa paste and drizzle with a little oil. Season. Bake at 325°F for 20 to 25 minutes, till cooked through and the juices run clear. Cover with foil if the edges of the chicken threaten to burn before the fillet is cooked. Serve with 3 tablespoons couscous (simply add boiling water according to package instructions), combined with sliced scallion (green onion), tomato, and cucumber, and chopped flat-leaf parsley and mint.

NB

CHICKEN PROVIDES SOME IMPORTANT B VITAMINS, AND ITS PROTEIN AIDS SATIETY.

LEMON-SCENTED STICKY CHICKEN WITH ROASTED VEGGIES

CALORIE COUNT: 287

The kids adore this—and it makes a light alternative to a traditional roast with all the big-boy trimmings. The idea is to fling everything into a pan and go away while the heat works its magic on the sweet lemon, and the chicken settles down to bless the vegetables with juice and flavor (a really good chicken is imperative). Just keep an eye on the pan to be sure that the vegetables at the edge aren't blackening too much. Otherwise, it's simply a case of feet up, crossword out. You may, of course, miss the roast potatoes. No matter. Cook them another day.

Serves 4

2 red onions, peeled and quartered, or 8 shallots, peeled
1 yellow bell pepper and 1 red bell pepper, seeded and cut into chunks
8 plum tomatoes
1 eggplant, coarsely cubed
Salt and pepper
1 free-range chicken (about 4 pounds/1.8kg)
1 tablespoon olive oil
2 lemons, halved
A handful of fresh thyme sprigs
1 sprig rosemary

Preheat the oven to 350°F. Place the vegetables in a roasting pan and season. Place the chicken on top and rub the oil into the skin. Squeeze 1 lemon over the chicken and vegetables, and add the rind to the pan. Place the second lemon, a few thyme sprigs, and the rosemary in the cavity of the chicken. Coarsely chop the remaining thyme leaves and sprinkle over the skin. Roast for 1 hour, or till the juices run clear. Halfway through cooking, check that the vegetables are not burning around the edges and move them around in the pan, tucking them under the chicken if necessary. Remove the chicken from the oven and let rest for 5 minutes, allowing the vegetables to cool slightly (room temperature is fine). Carve and serve on a generous mound of the sticky, lemony, char-roasted vegetables.

NB

PEPPERS ARE A GREAT SOURCE OF VITAMIN C, VITAL IN THE MANUFACTURE OF COLLAGEN, AN IMPORTANT STRUCTURAL PROTEIN.

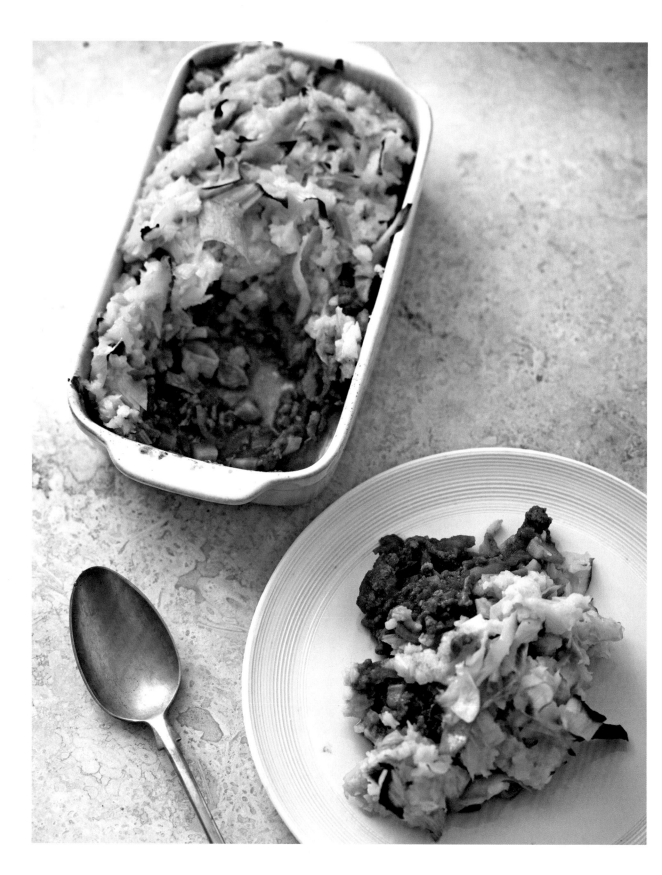

LIGHTWEIGHT COTTAGE PIE

CALORIE COUNT: 243

The pleasingly low calorie count here is achieved by swapping the usual topping of buttered mashed potatoes for a lighter celery root and leek lid, and using less meat than you normally would. The idea remains the same—a dish of unctuous loveliness to see you through a cold snap.

Serves 4

Spray oil
9 ounces/250g extra lean ground beef
1 large onion, diced
2 stalks celery, finely chopped
2 carrots, diced
One 14-ounce/400g can diced tomatoes
2 tablespoons tomato paste
1 tablespoon Worcestershire sauce
1 bay leaf
1 teaspoon fresh thyme leaves, chopped
Salt and pepper
1¼ cups/300ml boiling water
2 beef bouillon cubes
1 pound/500g celery root, peeled and cubed
½ cup/100g Vermont Creamery crème fraîche or fromage blanc
1 teaspoon peanut oil
2 young leeks, halved lengthwise and sliced in 2-inch lengths

Preheat the oven to 400°F. Spray a large pan with oil and brown the ground beef. Add the onion, celery, and carrots and cook for 10 minutes to soften. Stir in the tomatoes, tomato paste, Worcestershire, bay leaf, thyme, salt and pepper, water, and bouillon cubes. Bring to a boil, cover, and simmer for 30 minutes, stirring occasionally. Meanwhile, boil the celery root till very tender, drain, and mash with crème fraîche till as smooth as you wish. Heat the peanut oil in a pan and gently sauté the leeks. Add to the celery root mash and season well. Pour the beef into a shallow ovenproof dish, fish out the bay leaf, and top with the celery root mixture. Bake for 20 to 30 minutes, till the top is golden brown.

NB

USING CELERY ROOT FOR THE TOPPING INSTEAD OF POTATOES REDUCES THE CALORIES BY 75 PERCENT.

SARAH RAVEN'S CHICKEN PUTTANESCA

CALORIE COUNT: 247

British horticulturalist, kitchen gardener, food expert, and TV personality Sarah Raven is also a FastDiet fan. She says: "There is no need for your fast day meals to be punishing. This punchy puttanesca is low-fat and low-calorie but incredibly satisfying, and only needs a salad to make it a meal." Romaine lettuce would be a good choice.

Serves 6

1 tablespoon extra virgin olive oil
20 anchovy fillets, drained (fewer for a milder flavor)
4 cloves garlic, coarsely chopped
1 pound 5 ounces/600g cherry tomatoes (Sungolds give extra sweetness)
3 tablespoons good-quality mixed marinated pitted olives
2 tablespoons capers, rinsed and drained
12 skinless, boneless chicken thighs
Leaves from 1 small bunch fresh basil (about 1 ounce/30g)
Salt and pepper

Preheat the oven to 350°F. Heat the olive oil in a shallow, heavy casserole. Add the anchovies and garlic and gently cook for 2 to 3 minutes, till the anchovies have melted but the garlic has not browned. Add the tomatoes, olives, and capers, turn down the heat, and simmer gently. Add the chicken thighs and stir well to combine. Place the lid on the casserole and position on a middle shelf in the oven. Cook for 15 minutes. Remove from the oven and give the chicken a good stir so it's well coated in the juices. Return to the oven, uncovered, and cook for 20 minutes more. Allow to cool for a few minutes before stirring in the basil leaves. Taste for seasoning and serve.

NB

CHERRY TOMATOES CONTAIN LYCOPENE, AN ANTIOXIDANT THAT HELPS THE BODY FIGHT DISEASE.

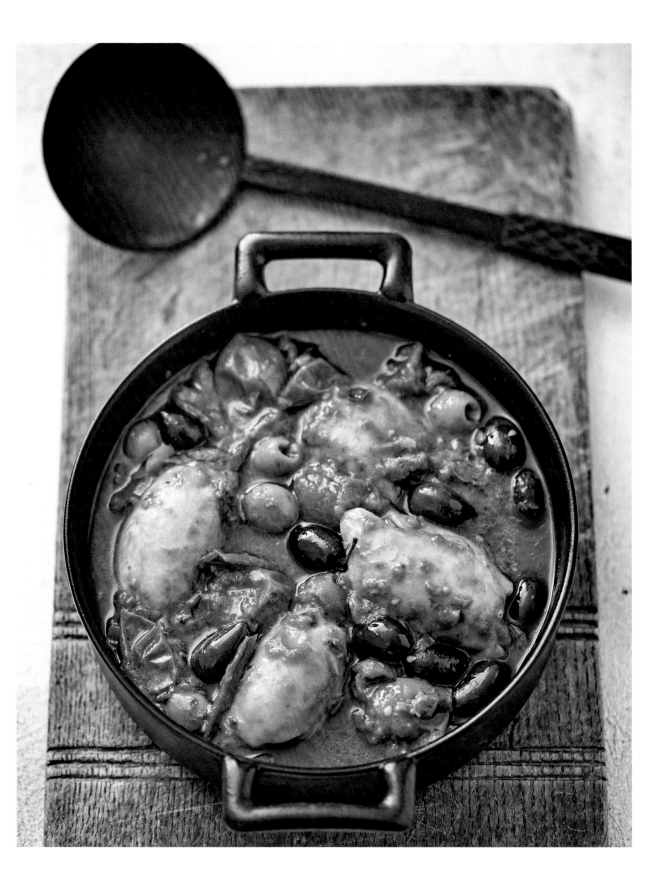

LO-LO MEATBALLS WITH CAVOLO NERO

CALORIE COUNT: 264

Lo-lo, because much of the saturated fat you'd usually find in a typical Italian mamma meatball has been stripped out by swapping in a leaner meat and eliminating all but the merest flash of oil. And the cavolo nero? Because it just sounds so great, the musketeer of the veggie world. Besides, cavolo nero—also known as Tuscan or black kale—is tasty, nutritious, easy to grow, and, yes, somehow *glamorous*.

Serves 2

Meatballs

7 ounces/200g lean ground pork or ground turkey
½ medium red onion, chopped
1 clove garlic, minced
1 small carrot, grated
A pinch of dried oregano
1 small egg, beaten
Salt and pepper
Spray oil, for the skillet

Tomato sauce

½ medium red onion, chopped
½ clove garlic, chopped

One 14-ounce/400g can diced tomatoes
Scant 2 ounces/50g fresh tomatoes, peeled
    (see page 15), seeded, and chopped
1 teaspoon tomato paste
A pinch of sugar
⅔ cup/200ml water
Red pepper flakes
A dash of Worcestershire sauce
1 teaspoon dried oregano

Cavolo nero

7 ounces/200g cavolo nero, steamed
A squeeze of lemon
Flaky sea salt

Combine the ground meat with the onion, garlic, carrot, oregano, egg, and salt and pepper. Mix well and shape into 12 small meatballs. In a skillet, brown gently over medium heat, about 4 minutes. For the sauce, sauté the onion till softened. Add the garlic and cook for 3 minutes more. Add the diced and chopped tomatoes, tomato paste, sugar, and water, plus red pepper and Worcestershire to taste. Simmer till reduced and unctuous. Add the meatballs and oregano, cover, and simmer for 20 minutes. Serve with steamed kale, dressed with a light squeeze of lemon and a scatter of flaky salt.

NB

PORK CONTAINS ZINC NEEDED FOR A HEALTHY IMMUNE SYSTEM, AND THIS DISH PROVIDES A THIRD OF YOUR RDA.

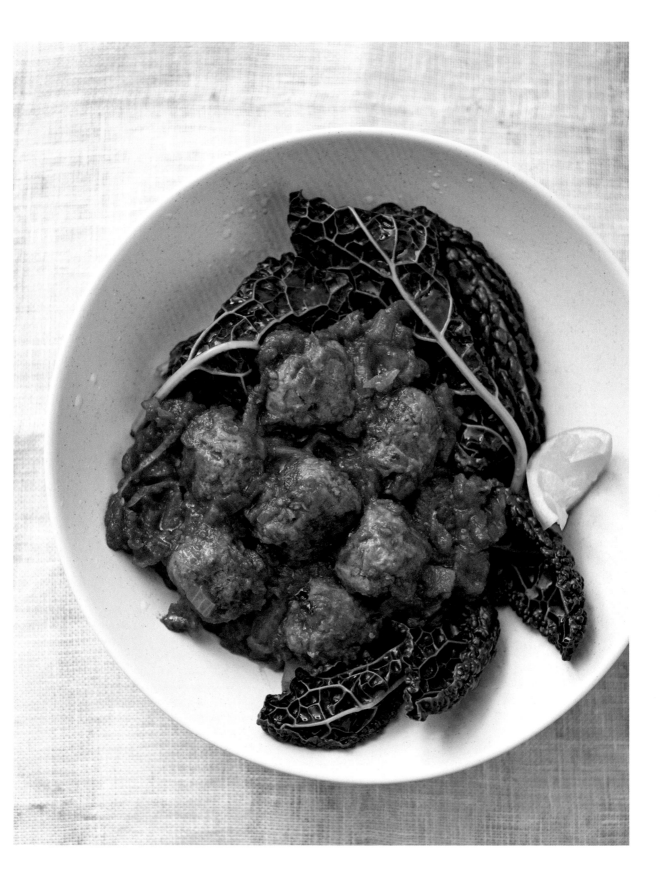

LETTUCE BOWLS WITH SHIITAKE MUSHROOMS AND HOISIN SHREDDED CHICKEN

CALORIE COUNT: 329

A fast day version of a Chinese standard, and perhaps one for a day when you're feeling frilly and creative. You could add a few chopped water chestnuts for extra crunch—they're barely a blip on the calorie radar.

Spray oil
1 teaspoon grated fresh ginger
1 teaspoon minced garlic
¼ head Chinese cabbage, shredded
1 carrot, julienned
Scant 2 ounces/50g oyster mushrooms, chopped
Scant 2 ounces/50g shiitake mushrooms, stemmed and chopped
Scant 2 ounces/50g bean sprouts
Ground white pepper
1 tablespoon hoisin sauce
1 cooked chicken breast, shredded
2 or 3 iceberg lettuce leaves
½ teaspoon toasted sesame seeds

Heat a wok and spray with oil. Add the ginger and garlic and stir-fry for 30 seconds. Add the cabbage, carrot, mushrooms, and bean sprouts. Stir-fry for 2 minutes, till the vegetables are just cooked but retain their bite. Season with pepper and add hoisin sauce. Add the shredded chicken and toss to mix. Place 2 or 3 iceberg lettuce leaves in a wide-rimmed cup, making a bowl effect. Spoon the chicken mixture into the bowl and serve with a scatter of toasted sesame seeds.

NB

EXOTIC MUSHROOMS CONTAIN ANTIOXIDANTS THAT GUARD AGAINST CELL DAMAGE AND HELP PREVENT TUMOR GROWTH.[1]

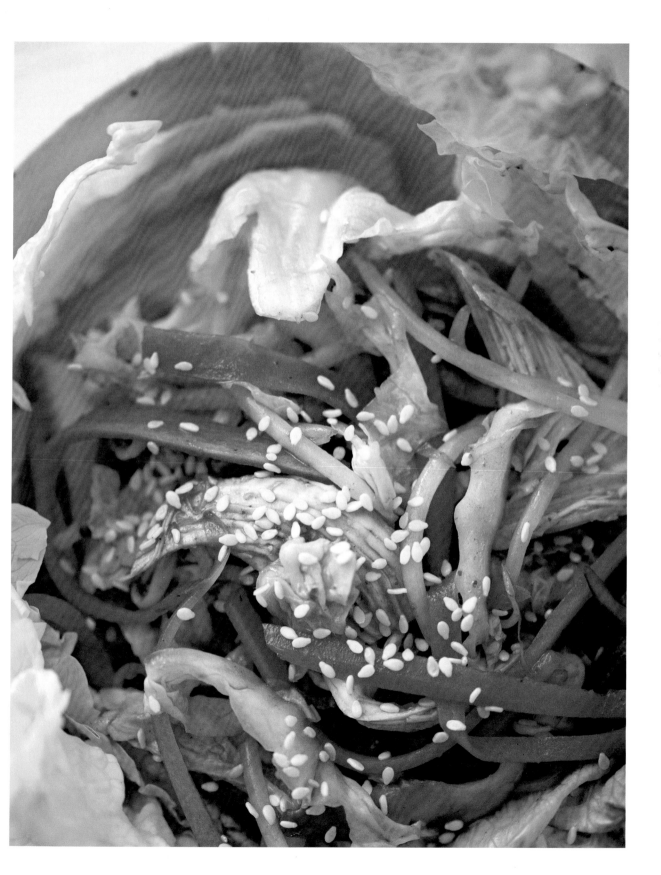

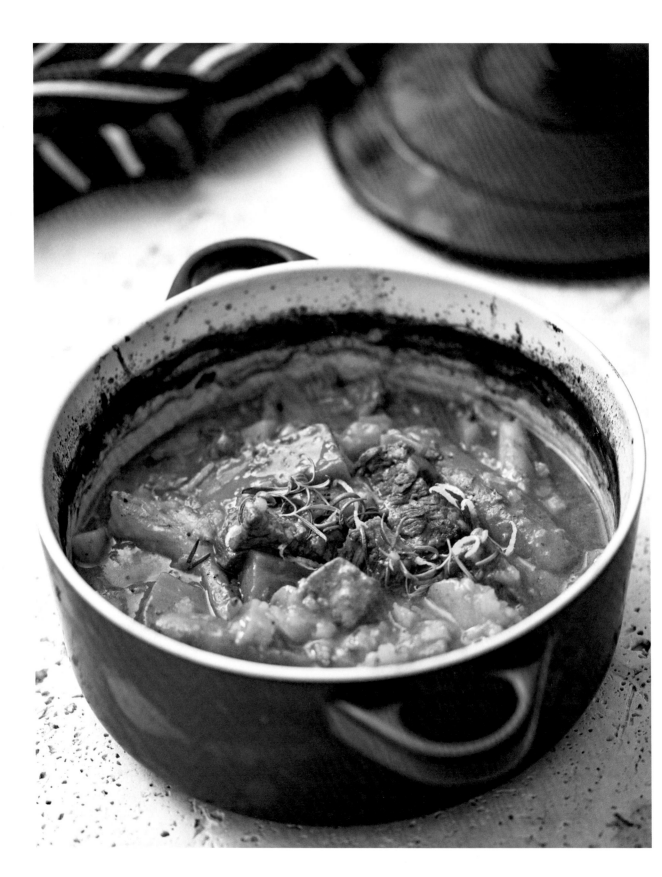

WARMING WINTER STEW

CALORIE COUNT: 385

Fast day food needn't be all about leaves and lemongrass. Here we've taken a classic and modified it to bump up the vegetables and lower the calories. On a nonfast day, you might have it with potatoes. But, really, it's a meal in itself without.

Serves 4

1 teaspoon olive oil
1 onion, diced
A handful fresh sage leaves
Salt and pepper
2 teaspoons all-purpose flour
14 ounces/400g stew beef or skirt steak, trimmed, cut into chunks
2 parsnips, peeled and quartered
4 carrots, halved crosswise
½ small butternut squash, seeded and coarsely chopped (no need to peel)
3 Jerusalem artichokes, peeled and halved
2 tablespoons tomato paste
1 bay leaf
1 cup/250ml red wine
1¼ cups/285ml vegetable stock
Grated shredded zest of 1 lemon and rosemary leaves, for garnish

Preheat the oven to 325°F. Heat the oil in a casserole, add the onion and sage leaves, and sauté for 3 minutes. Season the flour and dust the meat. Add to the casserole, along with the vegetables, tomato paste, bay leaf, wine, and stock. Stir gently and season. Bring to a boil, cover, place in the oven, and cook till the meat is tender and falls apart easily, about 3 hours. Garnish with lemon zest and a few rosemary leaves.

NB

THE VEGETABLES IN THIS STEW ARE LOW-GI, SO THEY WILL HELP REGULATE APPETITE.

THE GINGER MAN'S GRILLED CHICKEN

CALORIE COUNT: **291**

In my hometown of Brighton, England, one man really rules the restaurant roost: The Ginger Man. Ben McKellar is a local fixture, and we'd be lost without him. Here's his take on a chicken salad, modified for us fasters. It's the first time, incidentally, that The Ginger Man has ever concerned himself with calories when writing a recipe . . .

1 teaspoon finely chopped fresh ginger
2 tablespoons Asian fish sauce
A pinch of red pepper flakes
1 clove garlic, chopped
1 teaspoon agave nectar
Juice of 1 lime
2 tablespoons water
A little chopped fresh cilantro
1 skinless, boneless chicken breast (about 3½ ounces/100g)
3½ ounces/100g broccoli florets
4 teaspoons chopped peanuts

Mix the ginger, fish sauce, red pepper, garlic, agave, lime juice, water, and cilantro. Marinate the chicken in half of this mixture in the fridge for up to 6 hours. Steam the broccoli for 6 minutes and keep warm. Drain the chicken (discard the marinade), pat dry, and cook in a hot cast-iron skillet until done to your liking, perhaps 4 minutes on each side. Slice the chicken thinly, arrange on a plate with the broccoli, and drizzle the rest of the sauce over it. Sprinkle with the chopped peanuts and serve.

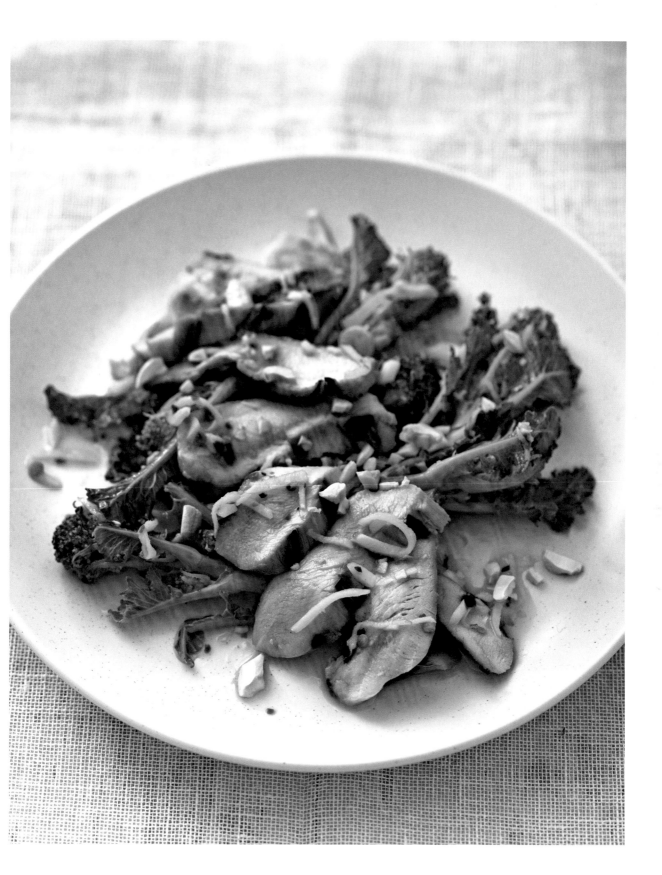

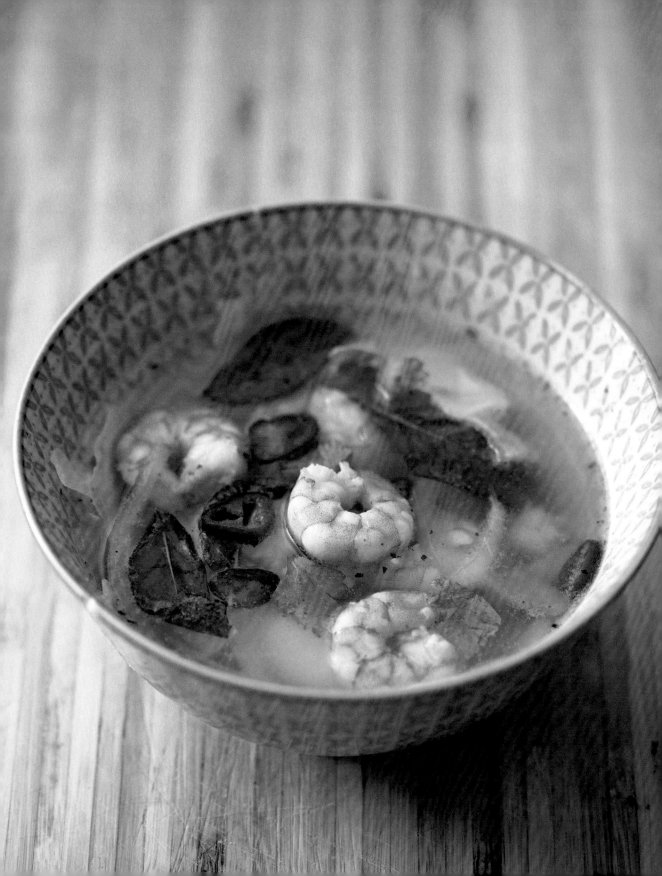

CHAPTER TEN

soups

FRAGRANT PHO

CALORIE COUNT: 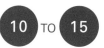 WITH SCANT 2 OUNCES/50G OF EXTRA VEGETABLES **10** TO **15**

Traveling in Laos and Vietnam, I came to adore the fresh, vivid taste of pho, served at every truck stop and roadside stall. This is a deliberately loose recipe. Add spring vegetables of your choosing. The quality of taste hinges on a good stock, so do contemplate making your own.

Serves 4

2 stalks lemongrass, outer leaves removed, inner stalk finely chopped
2 teaspoons grated fresh ginger
4 Kaffir lime leaves, torn
1½ quarts/1.5 liters vegetable stock
1 teaspoon palm sugar or light brown sugar
3 tablespoons Asian fish sauce
Juice of 1 lime
8 large shrimp, shelled and deveined
Fresh Thai basil, mint, and cilantro leaves and thinly sliced red chile, for serving

Use a mortar and pestle or a mini food processor to grind the lemongrass, ginger, and Kaffir lime leaves. Add to the stock in a large saucepan and boil for 10 minutes. Add sugar, fish sauce, and lime juice, tasting to check for balance. Cook shrimp in the broth till pink, 2 to 3 minutes. Add the herbs and red chile to serve.

To bulk up the broth, add snow peas, sugar snap peas, shredded spring cabbage, ribboned carrots, bean sprouts, shiitake mushrooms, or baby corn, along with the shrimp.

NB

EATING SOUP INCREASES SATIATION—AND STOPS YOU FROM OVEREATING.[1]

CLEAR TOFU BROTH

CALORIE COUNT: 54

Plenty of us crave clean, clear flavor on a fast day, and this tofu broth fits the bill. There's something vibrant and sparky about its combination of ginger, scallion, and cilantro. You somehow know instinctively that it is a Good Thing.

Serves 4

5 cups/1.2 liters vegetable stock
3½ ounces/100g shucked fresh baby corn
1 teaspoon julienned fresh ginger
3 scallions (green onions), finely chopped
3 teaspoons soy sauce
2 teaspoons mirin
1 teaspoon rice vinegar
8 ounces/225g tofu, diced
Scant 2 ounce/50g bean sprouts
Salt and pepper
Fresh cilantro leaves, for garnish

Heat the stock till boiling. Add the corn, ginger, and scallions. Simmer for 3 to 5 minutes. Add the soy sauce, mirin, vinegar, tofu, and bean sprouts, and season. Simmer for a minute more. Serve garnished with cilantro leaves.

NB

REGULAR CONSUMPTION OF GINGER MAY HELP REDUCE BODY WEIGHT.[2]

ROASTED RED PEPPER SOUP

CALORIE COUNT: 58

Roasting with a drizzle of olive oil will bring sweetness and intensity to peppers and tomatoes, at the limited cost of a few additional calories. You could cover the veggies for 10 minutes after roasting and then remove their skins, for a silkier soup.

Serves 4

3 large red bell peppers
3 ripe plum tomatoes, halved lengthwise
1 onion, quartered
3 cloves garlic, peeled
1 tablespoon olive oil
Salt and pepper
A pinch of sugar
1 teaspoon cumin seeds
Red pepper flakes
Juice and rind of ½ lemon
5 cups/1.2 liters chicken stock, plus more if needed
2 teaspoons tomato paste
1 teaspoon balsamic vinegar
Fresh basil leaves, for serving

Preheat the oven to 400°F. Place the bell peppers, tomatoes, onion, and garlic in a roasting pan. Drizzle with the oil; season with salt, pepper, the sugar, cumin, red pepper flakes to taste, and the lemon juice. Drop the lemon rind into the pan and roast till slightly caramelized, about 20 minutes. Remove the lemon rind and transfer everything else to a large saucepan. Add the stock and tomato paste. Bring to a boil and simmer for 10 minutes, removing any floating tomato skins. Puree in the pot with a stick blender, or carefully puree in batches in a canister blender. Add the vinegar, check seasoning, and puree till smooth. Add more stock if necessary to achieve the desired consistency. Reheat if necessary. Serve garnished with basil leaves.

NB

ROASTING THE PEPPERS HELPS RELEASE THE CAROTENOIDS; THE ADDITION OF OIL IMPROVES THEIR ABSORPTION INTO THE BODY.

RED VELVET SOUP

CALORIE COUNT: 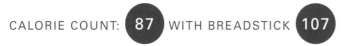 87 WITH BREADSTICK 107

A dense crimson broth for those soupy days when you want to do little more than curl up on the sofa and cuddle the cat.

Serves 4

1 tablespoon olive oil
1 onion, finely chopped
1 clove garlic, minced
A pinch of sugar
1 tablespoon tomato paste
2¼ pounds/1kg ripe red tomatoes, peeled
    and coarsely chopped

1 bay leaf
A few fresh thyme sprigs
2½ cups/600ml water
Salt and pepper
4 breadsticks, for serving

Heat the oil in a large saucepan and sauté the onion till soft but not browned. Stir in the garlic, sugar, tomato paste, and tomatoes. Add the bay leaf and thyme, tied together with kitchen twine for easy removal, and the water. Bring to a boil, then reduce to a simmer for 15 to 20 minutes. Remove the herbs and blend in the pot with a stick blender till smooth and velvety. Check the consistency, adding a little hot water if necessary. Reheat, season, and serve with a breadstick.

NB

TOMATOES CONTAIN SUBSTANCES THAT GUARD AGAINST CANCER, AND RESEARCH SUGGESTS THEY MAY ALSO HELP PREVENT NEURODEGENERATIVE DISEASES SUCH AS ALZHEIMER'S.[3]

SUMMERTIME SPECIAL SOUP

CALORIE COUNT: 91

Cooking with lettuce may not promise many thrills, but here its fresh green clarity, teamed with that of the cucumber and trumped by the glory of fresh shelled peas, works wonders. Frozen peas are fine. This cold soup is just the thing to eat as spring gets under way and the afternoons start to lengthen.

Serves 4

1 teaspoon vegetable oil
4 scallions (green onions), chopped
1 head lettuce (iceberg or Boston), shredded
1 large seedless cucumber, peeled, cored, and coarsely chopped
5 ounces/150g shelled fresh or frozen peas

1 quart/1 liter vegetable stock
1 vegetable bouillon cube
Salt and pepper
Minced chives, for serving
1 tablespoon crème fraîche or fromage blanc

Heat the oil in a large saucepan and add the scallions. Cook gently for 3 minutes. Add the lettuce, cucumber, and peas, stir, and sweat for 5 minutes. Add the stock and bouillon cube, season, and bring to a boil. Reduce heat and simmer, covered, for 15 minutes. Cool and puree in the pot with a stick blender. Refrigerate till cold. Check and adjust the seasoning and consistency. Serve with chives and a swirl of crème fraîche.

NB

FROZEN PEAS OFTEN CONTAIN MORE VITAMIN C THAN WEEK-OLD FRESH PEAS; FREEZING JUST AFTER PICKING LOCKS IN THE VITAMIN, WHICH OTHERWISE DECLINES OVER TIME.

CARROT AND GINGER SOUP

CALORIE COUNT: 93

Very low in calories, very pretty, very been-there-done-that—till you bring in star anise, cinnamon, cumin, and ginger. Then? *Ka-pow*.

Serves 2

1 onion, diced
1 teaspoon sunflower oil
1 star anise pod
1 teaspoon grated fresh ginger
3½ ounces/100g carrots, grated

½ cinnamon stick
2½ cups/600ml vegetable stock
Cumin seeds and fresh cilantro leaves, for serving

Sweat the onion in the oil in a saucepan with the star anise and ginger. Add the carrots, cinnamon, and stock and simmer for 15 to 20 minutes. Remove the star anise and cinnamon and puree the soup in the pot with a stick blender. Serve with a scattering of cumin seeds and fresh cilantro leaves.

NB

THERE IS GROWING EVIDENCE THAT CINNAMON HELPS CONTROL BLOOD SUGAR LEVELS.[4]

BLOODY MARY SOUP

CALORIE COUNT: 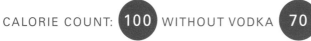 WITHOUT VODKA

This is an explosive tomato soup—packed with spiky flavor and (if you want) a jolt of vodka. It is served hot, with the usual Bloody Mary accompaniments of lemon, celery, and Tabasco and Worcestershire sauces. Ditch the vodka, of course, to cut back on fast day calories.

Serves 4

2¼ pounds/1kg ripe tomatoes, peeled and halved
2 red chiles, halved and seeded
Salt and pepper
½ teaspoon sugar
1½ teaspoons olive oil
1 quart/1 liter vegetable stock
1 tablespoon tomato paste

1 teaspoon bottled horseradish sauce
1 tablespoon Worcestershire sauce
1 tablespoon dry sherry
¼ cup vodka (optional)
Tabasco sauce, cracked black pepper, celery salt, celery stalks with leaves, and lemon slices, for garnish

Preheat the oven to 400°F. Place tomato halves and chiles in a roasting pan. Sprinkle with salt, pepper, and the sugar, drizzle with the oil, and bake till softened, about 20 minutes. Puree in a blender, adding a little stock to loosen. Transfer to a saucepan and stir in the remaining stock and the tomato paste. Heat through without boiling. Add the horseradish sauce, Worcestershire, sherry, and vodka (if using). Check and adjust the seasoning. Serve in heatproof glasses, with Tabasco, cracked black pepper, celery salt, celery stalks, and lemon slices. This also works as a cold soup.

NB

CELERY IS SAID TO HAVE "NEGATIVE CALORIES": ONE STICK CONTAINS ABOUT 2 CALORIES, BUT THE ENERGY COST OF EATING AND DIGESTING IT FAR OUTWEIGHS THIS.

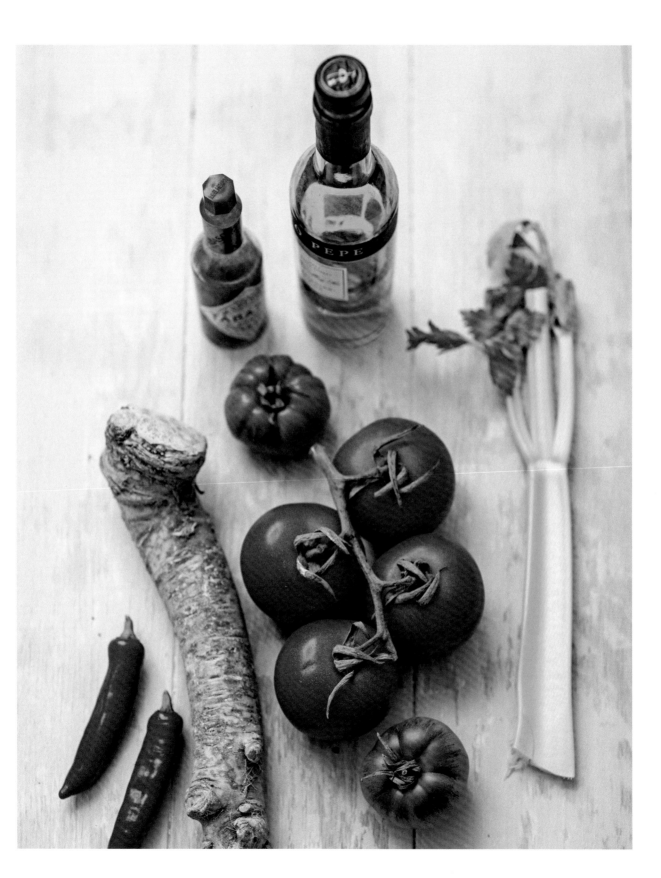

NORTH AFRICAN SPRING VEGETABLE BROTH

CALORIE COUNT: 102

This delicious clear soup is inspired by *Moro*, one of the most thumbed-through (and sauce-stained) cookbooks on my kitchen shelf. British chefs Sam and Sam Clark (Samuel and Samantha) have long used the flavors of Iberia and North Africa to great effect; the point here is a simple melody of taste, transferred from morning market to piping-hot soup bowl without much to-do. I've added sumac for a lemony kick (see Resources at the back of the book to find a source).

Serves 4

5¼ cups/1.25 liters chicken stock (homemade will give the best flavor
    to such an elegant soup)
5 ounce/150g fava beans, shelled, blanched, and peeled
5 ounces/150g fresh or frozen green peas
6 asparagus spears, trimmed and cut into ¾-inch pieces
2 globe artichokes, trimmed, quartered, chokes removed, very thinly sliced
A generous handful of fresh mint, flat-leaf parsley, and cilantro, chopped
2 scallions (green onions), finely chopped
1 tablespoon sumac
Juice of ½ lemon
Salt and pepper
4 thin rye crispbreads, for serving

Bring the stock to a gentle simmer in a large saucepan. Add the beans, peas, asparagus, and artichokes. Cook for 2 minutes, till tender. Remove from the heat and add the herbs, scallions, sumac, and lemon juice. Season carefully (sumac can be salty). Serve in white bowls with shards of broken crispbreads.

NB

THIS SOUP PROVIDES RESPECTABLE AMOUNTS OF POTASSIUM, MAGNESIUM, IRON, AND ZINC, AS WELL AS THE VITAMINS FOLATE, NIACIN, A, AND C.

SPINACH, SORREL, AND NUTMEG SOUP

CALORIE COUNT: 102 WITH A POACHED EGG 177

Now we're talking: a glorious, nutritious bowl of jolly green goodness that is, if such a thing were possible, the FastDiet distilled into a single spoonful. Try to find sorrel if you can (it's easy to grow, or find it at your local farmers' market or Whole Foods); it lends an acidic tang here and is well worth the search. If you have spare calories floating around, pop a poached egg on top (page 14) and marvel at your delightful bowl of good green gold.

Serves 4

1 tablespoon olive oil
1 onion, diced
1 clove garlic, minced
5¼ cups/1.25 liters chicken or vegetable stock
½ teaspoon chopped fresh ginger
A grating of nutmeg
Salt and pepper
1 pound/500g young spinach leaves
4½ ounces/125g sorrel leaves
2 tablespoons crème fraîche or fromage blanc
Fresh thyme leaves, for serving

Heat the oil in a large saucepan and sauté the onion and garlic till softened but not colored. Add the stock, ginger, and nutmeg to taste, and bring to a boil. Season and simmer for 10 minutes. Add the spinach and sorrel, and cook for 2 minutes more. Remove from the heat and stir in the crème fraîche. Adjust the seasoning, check consistency, and garnish with thyme leaves.

NB

NUTMEG CONTAINS A SUBSTANCE CALLED MACELIGNAN, WHICH CAN HELP PROTECT TEETH AGAINST CAVITIES.[5]

If you can't find sorrel, dandelion leaves work well, too; they'll give the soup a slight bitter edge.

EVERYTHING-FROM-THE-GARDEN SOUP

CALORIE COUNT: **108**

This is a glut in a bowl, and as such, defies rules. My only suggestion would be to try it semismooth—half of it fully blended, the other left chunky, then recombined prior to serving. It makes for an engaging texture, and one that promises to fill you up as soon as you look at it. The smoked paprika, too, adds a cunning twist.

Serves 4

1 tablespoon olive oil
1 pound/500g nonstarchy vegetables of your choice (zucchini, spinach, peppers,
   curly kale, Tuscan kale, leeks—whatever you have a glut of, or whatever is cheap
   and plentiful in the shops)
14 ounces/400g tomatoes, peeled and coarsely chopped
1 large onion, chopped
2 carrots, chopped
2 stalks celery, chopped
2 cloves garlic, minced
1 teaspoon smoked paprika
6¼ cups/1.5 liters vegetable stock (preferably homemade)
Salt and pepper
Fresh herbs of choice—perhaps chervil, marjoram, and/or thyme

Heat the oil in a large saucepan, add the vegetables, tomato, onion, carrots, celery, garlic, and smoked paprika, and sweat for 5 minutes. Add the stock, season, and simmer gently for 20 minutes. Cool slightly, then puree half of the soup in a blender, or with a stick blender, keeping the remaining half as it is. Recombine and reheat, stirring to achieve a semismooth soup. Serve topped with a tangle of herbs from the garden.

NB

THE ONLY NUTRIENT MISSING FROM THIS SOUP IS VITAMIN B_{12}—AND THAT'S JUST BECAUSE IT'S FOUND ONLY IN ANIMAL PROTEINS.

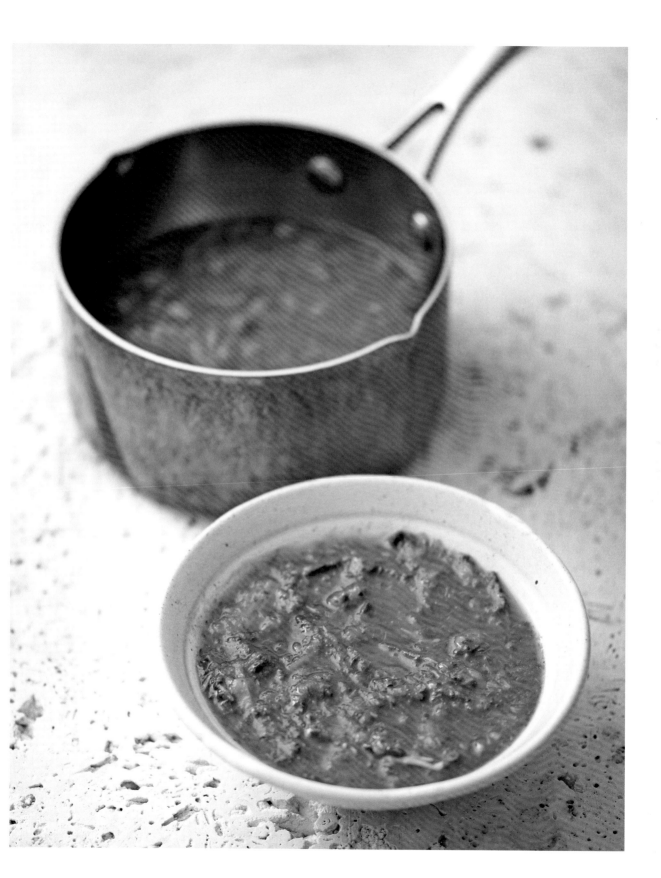

SPANISH GAZPACHO

CALORIE COUNT: 113

This is about as simple as soup can be—the very essence of summer, served fridge-cold and packed with wonderful flavor, impeccable nutritional value, and very few calories. This recipe is a classic version, given to me by my Pilates teacher Ana, who grew up in Spain. The original recipe dates from Roman times, and contained bread. You don't need it. You could try this with different colors and varieties of tomato—organic heirloom varieties may have more flavor than modern varieties.

Gazpacho does not freeze, so make this on the day and serve fresh.

Serves 2

1 red bell pepper, seeded and coarsely chopped
10 ounces/300g red tomatoes, ideally a mix of varieties, plus more diced for garnish
½ seedless cucumber, cored and coarsely chopped (5 to 7 ounces/150 to 200g),
    plus more diced for garnish
1 red chile, seeded and coarsely chopped
1 clove garlic, peeled
2 scallions (green onions), sliced, plus more for garnish
2 tablespoons red wine vinegar
1 tablespoon good-quality olive oil
6 ice cubes (optional)
Salt and pepper

Put the bell pepper, tomatoes, cucumber, chile, garlic, and scallions in a food processor and puree till smooth. Add the vinegar and olive oil, and quickly blend again to combine. To serve immediately, blend in the ice cubes; otherwise refrigerate till very cold. Check and adjust the seasoning. Serve cold with garnish.

NB

CAPSAICIN, THE ACTIVE INGREDIENT IN CHILE, HAS BEEN SHOWN TO INCREASE ENERGY EXPENDITURE AND IMPROVE SATIETY.[6]

For a fiery roasted gazpacho, first oven-roast the bell pepper, tomatoes, and chile, sprinkled with 2 teaspoons paprika. Allow to cool and blend with other ingredients as above.

Gazpacho plus . . . To make a heartier meal and include protein, serve gazpacho with

- a sprinkle of crabmeat and lemon zest (add 40 calories for scant 2 ounces/50g crab)

- or a crumble of feta and chopped black olives (add 25 for scant 1 ounce/25g olives and 100 for 1 ounce/30g feta)

- or with a chopped hard-boiled small egg (add 75) and a pinch of coarse sea salt

---

GREEN GAZPACHO

CALORIE COUNT: **277**

This is a cool alternative to traditional gazpacho, especially if you're not overly fond of tomatoes.

Serves 2

1 stalk celery (including leaves), coarsely chopped
1 small green bell pepper, seeded and coarsely chopped
½ seedless cucumber, peeled, cored, and chopped
½ avocado, chopped
1 fresh green chile (or less, to taste), chopped
1 teaspoon Tabasco sauce
2 garlic cloves, peeled

½ teaspoon sugar
3½ ounces/100g baby spinach leaves
1 ounce/30g walnuts
A handful of fresh basil leaves
A handful of fresh curly parsley
2 tablespoons sherry vinegar
1 tablespoon olive oil
1 tablespoon unflavored low-fat yogurt
4 ice cubes
1 cup/250ml water
Salt and pepper

Blitz all the ingredients in a blender, including the ice cubes. Add the water in stages, using more or less to achieve the desired consistency. Season and serve.

NB

AFTER OILY FISH, WALNUTS ARE THE NEXT-HIGHEST SOURCE OF LONG-CHAIN OMEGA-3 FATS.

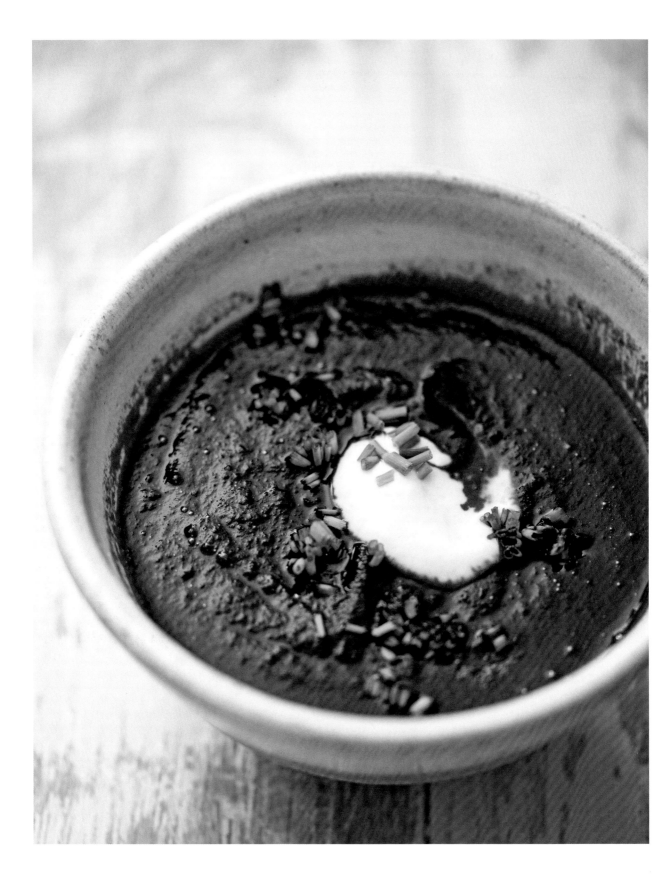

BEET AND APPLE SOUP WITH HORSERADISH

CALORIE COUNT: 116

The idea for this tangy autumn soup came from my friend Alex Renton, who made it for me one chilly lunchtime at his home in Edinburgh. I loved it so much that I made it for chef Allegra McEvedy, who asked to use it in her *Guardian* column, and now it's turning up here, a triumph of recipe recycling. This is the fast day version—no butter for sweating the onion, a swirl of yogurt instead of cream—but it's no less tasty than the original. It freezes like a dream, so you could double the recipe and have it handy as the nights lengthen.

Serves 4

1 pound/500g beets, trimmed and scrubbed but not peeled
1 tablespoon olive oil
2 onions, coarsely chopped
2 McIntosh apples, peeled, quartered, and cored, with a squeeze of lemon
    to prevent discoloration
6¼ cups/1.5 liters light chicken or vegetable stock
2 star anise pods
Salt and pepper
Minced chives
1 tablespoon unflavored low-fat yogurt
1 teaspoon bottled horseradish sauce

Preheat the oven to 400F. Place the beets in a small baking pan in ½-inch-deep water. Cover tightly with foil. Bake for an hour, or till a knife meets with little resistance. Take them out and run under cold water for a couple of minutes, till cool enough to peel.

Heat the oil in a heavy-bottomed saucepan. Add the onions, cover, and sweat over medium heat without coloring. Add the apples. Coarsely chop the peeled beets and add to the pan. Pour in the stock, add the star anise, season, and simmer for 15 minutes. Remove the star anise, then puree the soup in the pot with a stick blender. Serve with minced chives and a swirl of yogurt mixed with the horseradish sauce.

NB

BEETS CONTAIN DIETARY NITRATE, WHICH MAY HELP TO IMPROVE EXERCISE PERFORMANCE.[7]

SHIITAKE NOODLE DASHI

CALORIE COUNT: 137

This soup starts with a simple dashi—a Japanese stock that can be used as a base for countless soups. In Japan, sea vegetables are the heart of many dishes, but they're something we tend to ignore in the West. This is a shame, as seaweed in all its many forms is high in minerals, including iodine, potassium, calcium, and iron. And it's low in calories, of course. Dashi-kombu is sun-dried and cut into various sizes, then soaked to unlock the kelp's unique umami flavor. Rinse it first to wash away the salt of the drying process.

Dashi stock

3 slices kombu seaweed (about 4 inches long)
3¼ cups/750ml water
5 dried shiitake mushrooms

Soup and garnish

1½ cups/350ml dashi stock
3½ ounces/100g fresh shiitake mushrooms, stemmed and sliced

3½ ounces/100g rinsed shirataki noodles
1 teaspoon soy sauce
1 teaspoon mirin
½ teaspoon wasabi paste, or to taste
1 teaspoon finely julienned fresh ginger
1 scallion (green onion), finely chopped

To make the dashi stock, place the kombu in the water and slowly bring to a simmer for about 10 minutes; do not allow to boil. Remove the kombu, add the dried mushrooms, and boil for 1 minute, then turn off the heat and allow to sit, uncovered, for 20 minutes. Discard the mushrooms. If storing the dashi for later use, it will keep for up to 5 days in the fridge, and freezes well.

Bring the dashi stock to a simmer in a pan, and add the fresh mushrooms, noodles, soy sauce, mirin, wasabi (to taste), and ginger. Heat through and add the scallion to serve.

NB

KELP IS AN ASTONISHING PROVIDER OF CALCIUM—OVER A GRAM PER 3½ OUNCES.

SKIPPER'S SOUP

CALORIE COUNT: **142** WITH YOGURT **152**

A quick-fix, morale-boosting soup from British food writer, seafarer, and friend Alex Renton. This, he says, is smoky, spicy, and full of fiber—great for cold days or after exercise, and easy to rustle up from cupboard ingredients, even in the galley belowdecks while a storm rages outside. It freezes well, so it makes sense to make a quantity and keep it in portion sizes. "I always prefer homemade stock, though the calorie count will be higher than with a bouillon cube," he adds. "But if you strain and chill the homemade stock after making it, you can remove much of the fat." Aye aye, skipper.

Scant 1 ounce/25g good-quality Spanish chorizo
1 small onion, finely chopped
7 ounces/200g canned white, cannellini, or butter beans, or chickpeas, drained
1¼ cups/300ml chicken stock
A pinch of smoked paprika
Salt and pepper
1 tablespoon unflavored low-fat yogurt, for serving (optional)

Chop the chorizo into small chunks and heat gently in a heavy-bottomed saucepan. When it has released some fat, add the onion and fry gently till softened. Add the beans and stock and simmer for 10 minutes. Puree in the pot with a stick blender till smooth. Add the paprika, check the seasoning, and serve. Top with a dollop of low-fat yogurt if you can spare the calories.

NB

THE FIBER CONTENT HERE IS 7G PER PORTION, OVER A THIRD OF YOUR RECOMMENDED DAILY AMOUNT.

SKINNY BOUILLABAISSE

CALORIE COUNT: 163

My sister Debs is incredibly skilled in the kitchen, having trained in the world-renowned kitchens at Ballymaloe in Ireland. This soup is designed to bring all the rounded, rich flavor of a traditional French fish stew to your low-calorie fast day soup bowl. Even without the usual butter, aioli, and croutons, this is still quite a fancy dish. One to make when your Fast friends drop by. Notice the calorie count. Sing.

Serves 4

1½ teaspoons olive oil

1 onion, thinly sliced

1 bulb fennel, trimmed and thinly sliced

4 cloves garlic, minced

1 teaspoon grated fresh ginger

1 red chile, finely chopped (seed first if you prefer less heat)

A generous pinch of saffron threads

1 teaspoon sweet paprika

One 14-ounce/400g can diced tomatoes

5¼ cups/1.25 liters fish or vegetable stock

½ teaspoon sugar

1 bay leaf

Salt and pepper

14 ounces/400g white fish fillet, cut into chunks

8 mussels, scrubbed

8 large raw shrimp, peeled and deveined, tails left on

A handful of fresh flat-leaf parsley, chopped

Lemon juice, for serving

Heat the olive oil in large heavy-bottomed saucepan over medium heat. Add the onion and fennel and cook, stirring occasionally, for about 5 minutes, till softened but not colored. Add the garlic, ginger, chile, saffron, and paprika and cook for 2 minutes more, till fragrant. Stir in the tomatoes, stock, sugar, and bay leaf, scraping the pan with a wooden spoon to release any stickiness on the base. Season and simmer for 20 to 25 minutes. Gently lower the fish, mussels, and shrimp into the soup, cover the pan, and cook for 2 to 3 minutes till the fish and shrimp are just opaque and the mussels have opened (discard any that have failed to open). Check the seasoning and serve with a scattering of parsley and a squeeze of lemon juice to taste.

NB

ONLY 2G FAT, BUT A SUBSTANTIAL FULL OUNCE OF PROTEIN PER SERVING—AND A TON OF TASTE.

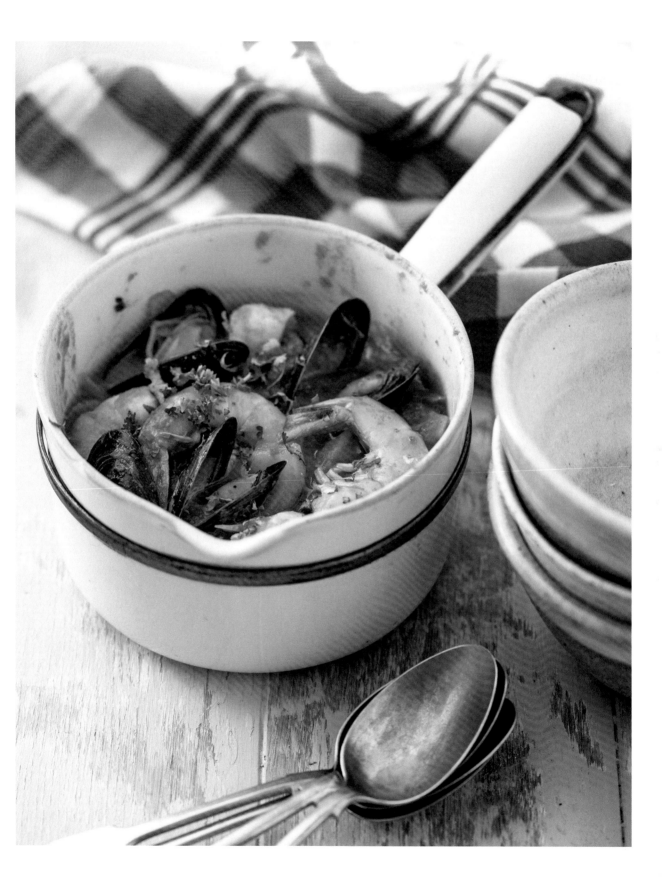

FAST DAY MINESTRONE

CALORIE COUNT: 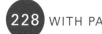 228 WITH PASTA 313

Minestrone literally means "big soup"—and that's exactly what you'll get from this recipe. This is the heartland of FastDiet cooking: filling but full of sunny flavor and packed with vital vitamins. The vegetables in a minestrone can, of course, vary according to your preference and what's in season. Try curly kale instead of spinach, asparagus instead of green beans, and chickpeas or favas instead of cannellini, or throw in a handful of frozen peas toward the end of cooking. For speed and simplicity, you could simply add handfuls of frozen vegetables to your broth—peas, corn kernels, carrots, broccoli. Sacrifice the pasta if you want to save on calories and GL. For minestrone verde, leave out the tomatoes, stick to green veggies, and bump up the stock by 100ml/scant ½ cup.

Serves 4

1 tablespoon olive oil	One 14-ounce/400g can diced tomatoes
1 onion, diced	5 ounces/150g cooked cannellini beans
1 clove garlic, chopped	3½ ounces/100g thin green beans,
3 stalks celery, chopped	chopped
1 small leek, diced	1 zucchini, diced
2 carrots, diced	3½ ounces/100g baby spinach leaves
1 quart/1 liter vegetable or chicken stock	Fresh oregano and basil leaves
1 chicken bouillon cube	Salt and pepper
1 bay leaf	2 teaspoons grated Parmesan, for serving
3½ ounces/100g small pasta, such as	
orecchiette or conchigliette	

Heat the oil in a large saucepan and sauté the onion and garlic till softened. Add the celery, leek, and carrots and cook for 3 to 4 minutes more, till golden and flavorful. Add the stock, bouillon cube, and bay leaf, and bring to a boil. Add the pasta, if using, and cook for 4 minutes. Reduce the heat and add the tomatoes, cannellini beans, green beans, and zucchini. Simmer for 2 to 4 minutes (depending on the cooking time of your chosen pasta), then add the spinach leaves, herbs, and seasoning. Serve with a little Parmesan and more fresh herbs.

NB

IF YOU WANT A LITTLE CARBOHYDRATE BUT FEWER CALORIES, SWAP THE PASTA FOR POTATO, WHICH WILL ADD ONLY 18.

DEBS'S CHICKEN NOODLE SOUP WITH AVOCADO AND CUCUMBER

CALORIE COUNT: 237

This is my sister's take on the classic chicken noodle soup, beloved of mums everywhere. The addition of cucumber, avocado, and lime makes for a novel spoonful. Truly a chicken noodle soup for the soul.

Serves 4

3½ ounces/100g rice noodles
5½ cups/1.25 liters homemade chicken stock
A pinch of red pepper flakes or finely chopped fresh chile
2 skinless, boneless chicken breasts, thinly sliced (about 7 ounces/200g)
Salt and pepper
A pinch of sugar
½ head iceberg lettuce, shredded
½ seedless cucumber, cored and diced
1 avocado, diced, with a squeeze of lemon to prevent discoloration
2 scallions (green onions), thinly sliced
2 tablespoons coarsely chopped fresh cilantro
Lime wedges, for serving

Cook the noodles according to package instructions, drain, refresh, drain again, and set aside. Bring the stock to a boil; add the red pepper and chicken. Reduce the heat, season, add the sugar, and simmer gently till the chicken is cooked, 4 to 5 minutes depending on the size of the chicken pieces. Divide the lettuce, cucumber, avocado, scallions, and cilantro among four hot soup bowls. Add the noodles to the hot broth, bring swiftly to a boil, and serve over the vegetables. Add a squeeze of lime.

NB

AVOCADOS ARE A GREAT SOURCE OF ANTIOXIDANT VITAMIN E, WHICH IS IMPORTANT FOR YOUR IMMUNE SYSTEM.

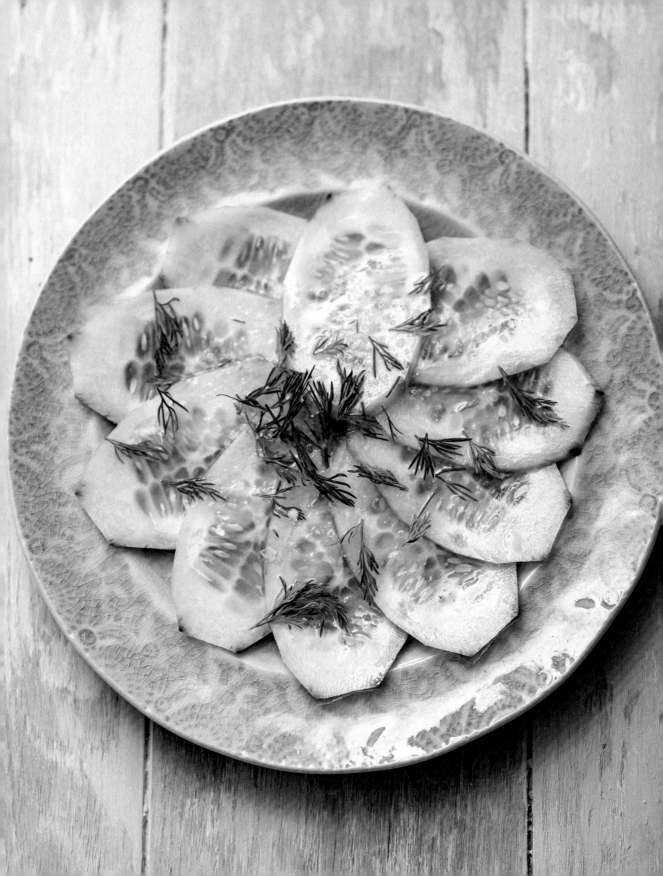

CHAPTER ELEVEN

salads

SUMMER CUCUMBER SALAD WITH DILL

CALORIE COUNT: 43

As simple a salad as was ever thrown together on a plate. It doesn't require fanfare, just a fork. Serve with whole baked fish, page 114.

Serves 4 as a side dish

1 large garden cucumber, peeled and thinly sliced

Dressing

1 tablespoon mild olive oil
2 teaspoons Dijon mustard
2 teaspoons white wine vinegar
1 teaspoon sugar
Salt and pepper

2 tablespoons chopped fresh dill

Place cucumber slices in a serving dish. Whisk the dressing ingredients and add, finishing with a good grind of black pepper. Sprinkle with the dill and serve.

NB

IN A CLINICAL TRIAL, PATIENTS WITH METABOLIC SYNDROME GIVEN DILL FOR 12 WEEKS SHOWED A REDUCTION IN BLOOD LIPIDS.[1]

FENNEL, CUCUMBER, AND RADISH SALAD WITH A CITRUS VINAIGRETTE

CALORIE COUNT: 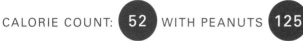 52 WITH PEANUTS 125

A star of Italian cooking, fennel is only just finding its way into our hearts. It's a humble thing, but full of nutrients. According to researchers, the "most fascinating phytonutrient compound in fennel" may be anethole—the primary component of its volatile oil. In animal studies, the anethole in fennel has repeatedly been shown to reduce inflammation and to help prevent the occurrence of cancer.[2] You needn't get too hung up on any of this, though. Just enjoy its sharp licorice flavor.

Serves 2

Dressing

1 teaspoon finely chopped lemongrass
1 teaspoon soy sauce
1 teaspoon sesame oil
3 teaspoons lime juice
A pinch of sugar

Salad

1 bulb fennel, very thinly sliced on a mandoline
½ seedless cucumber, halved lengthwise, cored, and thinly sliced into crescents
7 ounces/200g assorted radishes, trimmed and thinly sliced
1 scallion (green onion), finely chopped
½ teaspoon grated fresh ginger
Red pepper flakes, to taste
A handful of fresh cilantro and mint leaves
10 peanuts, chopped (optional)

Combine the dressing ingredients. Assemble the salad and dress. Add a handful of the chopped peanuts if your calorie budget allows.

NB

YOU'LL GET A QUARTER OF YOUR RDA OF POTASSIUM FROM THIS SALAD.

ASPARAGUS SALAD WITH RED ONION AND GRILLED MUSHROOM

CALORIE COUNT: 110

Anyone who understands and adores seasonal cooking will know the thrill of the first asparagus arriving. And asparagus contains only around 125 calories per pound, so it's fab as long as you don't treat it to a butter bath. Young asparagus may work best in this recipe, but don't overcook them. Treat as you would vermouth in a martini and barely show them the heat. In, out, eat.

Serves 4

1 tablespoon olive oil
2 red onions, cut into eighths
4 large portobello mushroom caps, sliced
3 cloves garlic, minced
3 zucchini, thick-sliced on the diagonal, blanched, and refreshed
10 ounces/300g young asparagus, trimmed, blanched, and refreshed
Salt and pepper
A squeeze of lemon
2 tablespoons grated or shaved Parmesan cheese

Heat the oil in a large cast-iron skillet. Add the onions and cook for 2 minutes. Add the mushrooms and grill till softened and charred, turning often. Add the garlic and zucchini and cook for 3 minutes more. Place on a platter and top with a mess of asparagus, thrown on like pick-up sticks. Season well, then add a squeeze of lemon and a generous sprinkling of Parmesan.

NB

THIS SUBSTANTIAL SALAD PROVIDES YOUR ENTIRE FOLATE REQUIREMENT FOR A DAY.

PENNY'S BEET SALAD

CALORIE COUNT: 114

My dear friend Penny is a world-class beet queen, and this salad—a fiery mouthful of cumin, OJ, horseradish, and mustard—is her pièce de résistance. The grating needs to be done on the biggest holes of the grater to prevent the whole event from turning to mush—take your time; it makes for a contemplative moment in a busy day. (Beet stems and leaves can, by the way, be eaten too, so don't chuck them. Save for another salad, or sauté with garlic in olive oil till just wilted—then sprinkle with Parmesan and crack out the black pepper.)

Serves 4

3 carrots, peeled and coarsely grated
½ celery root, trimmed, peeled, and julienned on a mandoline
3 medium beets, scrubbed and coarsely grated
1 apple, grated

Dressing

1 tablespoon grated horseradish
1 tablespoon good-quality olive oil
1 tablespoon orange juice
1 teaspoon prepared English mustard
1 clove garlic, minced
Salt and pepper

Garnish

1 teaspoon toasted cumin seeds, whole or ground
1 tablespoon pumpkin seeds (pepitas)
Fresh cilantro leaves, for serving

Assemble the vegetables and apple in a bowl. Combine the dressing ingredients, add to the bowl, and mix well. Serve scattered with seeds and cilantro leaves.

NB

SCIENTIFIC STUDIES SHOW THAT BEETS CAN HELP TO LOWER BLOOD PRESSURE.[3]

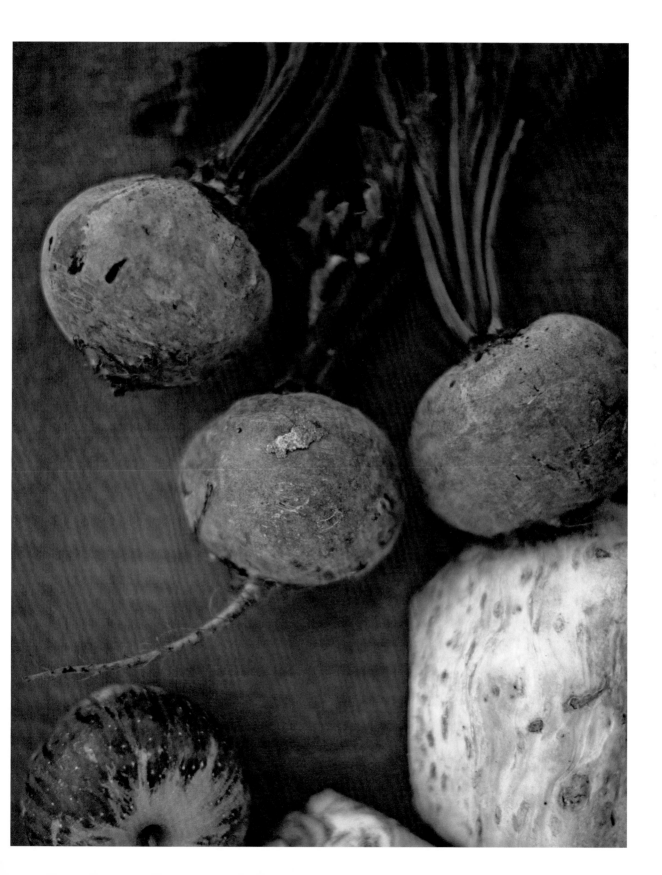

PEA, SHRIMP, AND PEA SHOOT SALAD

CALORIE COUNT: **152**

This is a wonderful springtime salad—pale green, pretty pink, and dancing with clean, fresh flavors. Glitz it up with fresh peas right out of the pod if you want something a bit posh.

Serves 2

Dressing

1 tablespoon good-quality olive oil
1 teaspoon white wine vinegar or tarragon vinegar
½ teaspoon Dijon mustard
Salt and pepper

Salad

3½ ounces/100g cooked shrimp, peeled and deveined
3½ ounces/100g frozen peas, thawed under hot running water
1 small head Bibb or Boston lettuce, leaves separated
Scant 2 ounces/50g pea shoots
1 scallion (green onion), thinly sliced
1½ tablespoons/15g fresh tarragon leaves
A handful of fresh mint leaves

Whisk together the dressing. (You can quadruple the quantities and keep the remaining dressing in the fridge for 3 to 4 days.) Assemble the salad ingredients and drizzle with dressing. Toss and serve.

NB

A PORTION OF THIS SALAD DELIVERS THE SAME AMOUNT OF IRON AS A SMALL STEAK, AND THE VITAMIN C WILL AID ITS ABSORPTION.

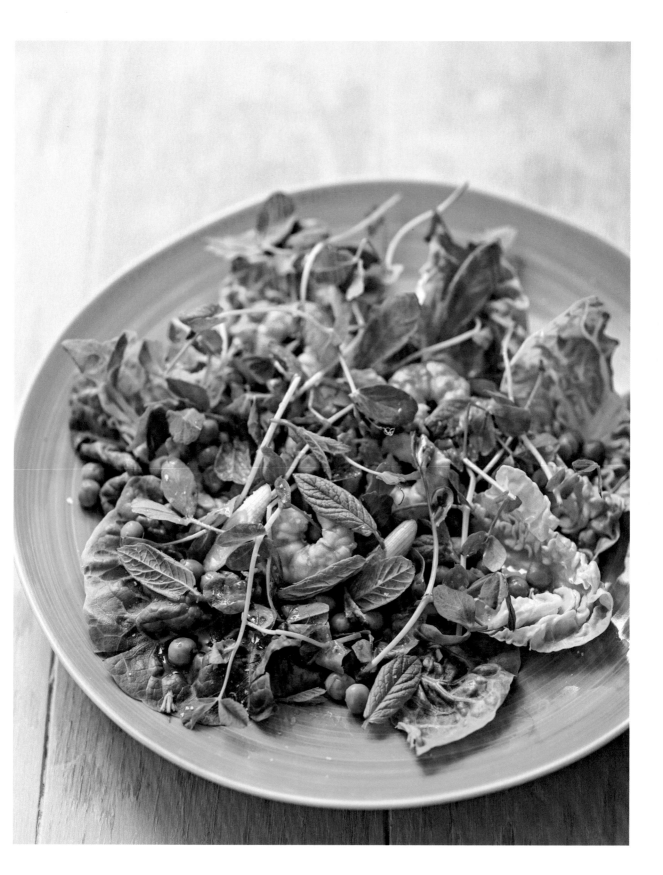

SPROUTS SPECTACULAR

CALORIE COUNT: **161**

Sprouts are glorious little things, full of nutrients and unexpected flavor. There are countless varieties—broccoli, alfalfa, clover, lentil, mustard, onion, mung, soybean, sunflower—but I'm particularly fond of radish sprouts, which have the pepper punch of radishes and look immensely appealing on the plate, a crazy tangle of filigree filaments to confuse your fork.

Serves 4

Dressing

1 tablespoon lime juice
A handful of fresh cilantro, finely chopped
1 teaspoon flaxseed oil
1 teaspoon sesame oil
½ teaspoon soy sauce
1 teaspoon grated fresh ginger
1 teaspoon honey
Salt and pepper

Salad

2 carrots, julienned
1 stalk celery, julienned
2 red apples, cored, thinly sliced, and tossed with a squeeze of lemon to prevent discoloration
7 ounces/200g mung bean sprouts
5 ounces/150g alfalfa sprouts
3½ ounces/100g radish sprouts
Scant 2 ounces/50g shelled sunflower seeds, for serving

Combine the dressing ingredients, remembering that the quantities are just a guideline. Assemble the salad, dress, and scatter with seeds.

NB

THERE IS PLENTY OF VITAMIN E AND A DECENT AMOUNT OF MAGNESIUM IN THIS SUPER HEALTHY SALAD.

SUPERFOOD BELLY BUSTER

CALORIE COUNT: 173

Much has been written about the towering promise of "superfoods"—and while they do tend to offer substantial nutritional advantage, there's also a bit of marketing puff in the mix. This salad brings together an all-star cast that delivers ample vitamins, minerals, and fiber.

Serves 4

Salad

3 tablespoons quinoa, cooked, drained, and cooled

3½ ounces/100g broccoli florets with stems, sliced, blanched, and refreshed

3½ ounces/100g green beans, cut into 1¼-inch lengths, blanched and refreshed

3½ ounces/100g frozen peas, thawed under hot running water

3½ ounces/100g baby arugula leaves

3½ ounces/100g baby spinach leaves

½ red onion, thinly sliced

3 ripe tomatoes, coarsely chopped

½ seedless cucumber, peeled, halved lengthwise, cored, and sliced into crescents

A handful of alfalfa sprouts

Juice of 1 lemon

1 tablespoon good-quality olive oil

Salt and pepper

Garnish

Plenty of chopped fresh mint and flat-leaf parsley

Lemon wedges

1 tablespoon mixed sesame and pumpkin seeds, lightly toasted

Pomegranate seeds

Mix the quinoa with the rest of the salad ingredients. Dress with the lemon juice and olive oil, and season. Serve the salad with chopped herbs, lemon wedges, and a scattering of sesame, pumpkin, and pomegranate seeds.

NB

QUINOA CONTAINS DOUBLE THE PROTEIN AND MAGNESIUM, 3 TIMES THE POTASSIUM AND ZINC, AND 7 TIMES THE IRON AND CALCIUM OF OTHER GRAINS SUCH AS BROWN RICE.

To make a more substantial meal, add a handful of crumbled feta (add 125 calories for scant 2 ounces/50g feta, 30 calories per serving).

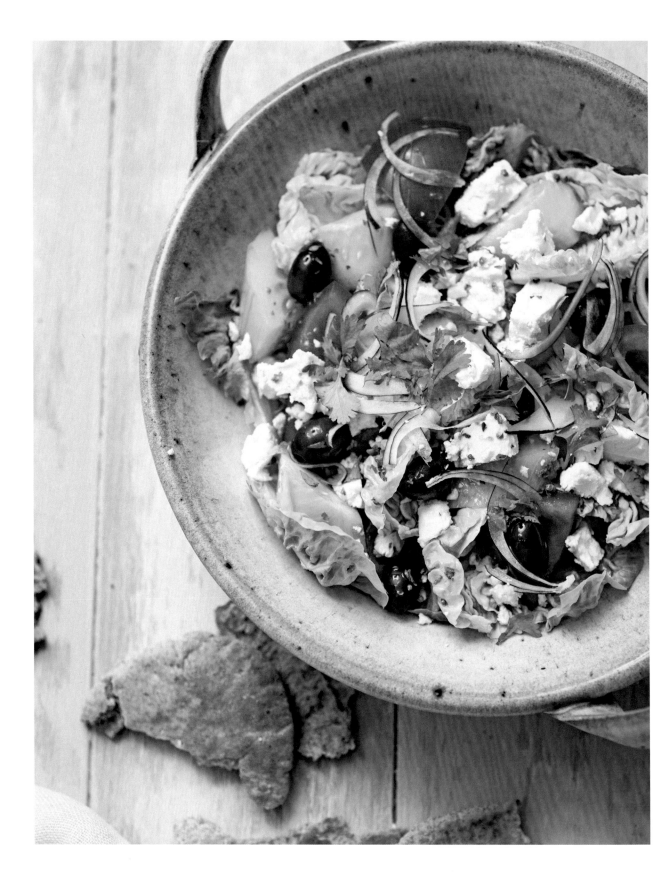

GREEK SALAD WITH OREGANO AND MINT

CALORIE COUNT: 229

If you want to eat dairy protein on a fast day, feta—traditionally made from sheep or goat milk—is a good choice, lower in calories than many other cheeses. It's strongly flavored, too, so you don't need much to feel its presence. It's worth going easy in any case, as feta is relatively high in salt.

To make the very best Greek salad, choose the finest tomatoes you can. I generally buy mine on the vine and ripen them on a sunny windowsill till they're bursting with flavor. Your best garden or farmers' market heirloom tomato is just the thing. A rock-hard, fridge-cold, anemic tomato from a plastic tray isn't even in the same ballpark.

Serves 4

Dressing

2 tablespoons good-quality olive oil
2 tablespoons red wine vinegar
A pinch of sugar
Juice of 1 lemon
A handful of each of fresh mint leaves and flat-leaf parsley, chopped
1 teaspoon dried oregano
Salt and pepper

Salad

14 ounces/400g best-quality ripe tomatoes, quartered and cored
1 red onion, very thinly sliced
1 seedless cucumber, peeled, cored, and cut into chunks
I small head romaine lettuce, leaves separated
12 kalamata olives
7 ounces/200g good-quality feta cheese, broken into pieces

Whole-grain pita, cut into strips and toasted, for serving

Whisk together the dressing. Assemble the salad, dress, and serve with hot pita fingers.

NB

FETA IS LOWER IN CALORIES THAN MOST OTHER WHOLE-MILK CHEESES—IT IS 20 PERCENT FAT, WHILE CHEDDAR IS 35 PERCENT. LOOK FOR TRADITIONAL FETA MADE FROM SHEEP'S MILK.

CALORIE COUNT: 231

Orange feta salad makes a great alternative: For 4 people, combine 2 heads endive, sliced crosswise; 1 small red onion, sliced; the segments of 2 oranges; 7 ounces/200g crumbled feta; and 12 pitted green olives. Dress with a vinaigrette made from the juice of 1 orange, 2 tablespoons olive oil, 2 tablespoons white wine vinegar, a pinch of sugar, and salt and pepper.

CALORIE COUNT: 312

Or try an Eastern feta salad for four, with 7 ounces/200g baby spinach leaves, 4 ripe tomatoes, 1 tablespoon toasted pine nuts, and 7 ounces/200g feta cheese. Dress with 2 tablespoons olive oil, fresh oregano, the juice of 1 lemon, 1 tablespoon red wine vinegar, a hint of garlic, salt and pepper, and a generous sprinkle of sumac, plus shards of 2 crisply toasted pitas.

SIMPLE HERB SALAD WITH WARM BUTTERED ALMONDS

CALORIE COUNT: 223

Fine ingredients will deliver deliciousness without too much effort, and this simple, simple salad of baby herb leaves is indeed a wonderful thing. Here, a nugget of unsalted butter is, to my mind, a worthwhile calorie cost—though you could simply add the coarsely chopped almonds without sautéing. Try this with Harissa-Spiked Chicken, page 148.

Serves 4 as a side dish

3½ ounces/100g whole almonds, skin on
2 teaspoons/20g unsalted butter
Coarse sea salt and cracked black pepper
Scant 2 ounces/50g baby arugula
3½ ounces/100g mixed fresh herbs (cilantro, flat-leaf parsley, dill, and tarragon)
Juice of 1 lemon
1 tablespoon good-quality olive oil

Lightly sauté the almonds in the butter for 5 minutes with a good seasoning of salt and pepper. Remove from the pan, drain on paper towels, then coarsely chop. Assemble the arugula and herb leaves, and toss gently with the lemon and olive oil. Scatter with the almonds and serve.

NB

GET HALF YOUR RDA OF VITAMIN C WITH THIS SIMPLE SIDE DISH.

WINTER WALDORF SALAD

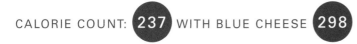

CALORIE COUNT: 237 WITH BLUE CHEESE 298

I love this take on the classic, first served at New York's Waldorf Astoria Hotel in 1893. This version is deliberately pink-cheeked, as if recently in from the cold. Go for red endive, red apple, and a quartered fig for prettiness. If you have calories to spare, you could add a hint of a blue cheese—perhaps a few crumbles of Stilton.

Serves 2

Salad

1 small head red endive (Treviso), leaves separated
1 head endive, sliced crosswise
1 red apple, cored, chopped, and tossed with a squeeze of lemon to prevent discoloration
2 stalks celery, chopped
Scant 2 ounces/50g broken walnut halves
1 fresh fig, cut into eighths

About 1 ounce/30g crumbled blue cheese (optional)

Dressing

2 tablespoons unflavored low-fat yogurt
1 teaspoon Dijon mustard
1 tablespoon lemon juice
Salt and pepper

Combine the salad ingredients in a bowl. Combine dressing and drizzle over the salad.

NB

PLENTY OF HEALTHY MONOUNSATURATED FAT AND VITAMIN E IN THIS SALAD.

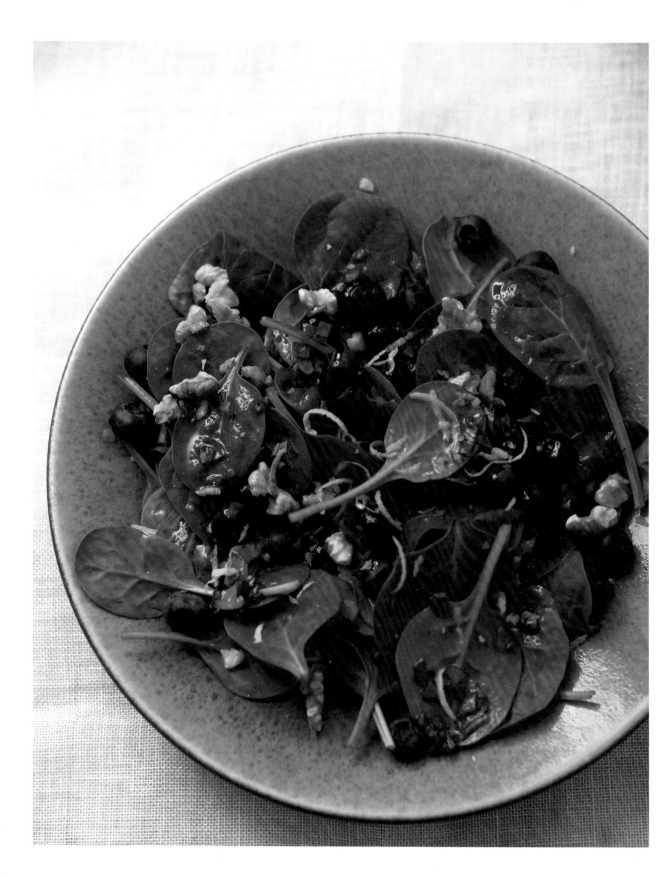

SPINACH, BLUEBERRY, AND WALNUT SALAD WITH A TARRAGON VINAIGRETTE

CALORIE COUNT: 239

I love the very idea of this salad—the pop of blueberries, the sweet tarragon, the rich crunch of walnut. It's something to toss together on a long, hot day. No mess, no fuss, just great.

Serves 2

Vinaigrette

2 teaspoons peanut oil
2 teaspoons cider vinegar
Zest of ½ lemon, in curls
1 tablespoon fresh tarragon leaves
Salt and pepper

Salad

7 ounces/200g baby spinach leaves
Scant 2 ounces/50g walnut halves, slightly broken
3½ ounces/100g fresh blueberries

Prepare the vinaigrette. Combine the spinach, walnuts, and blueberries and dress.

NB

EATING BLUEBERRIES SEEMS TO OFFER NEUROPROTECTION AGAINST SLOW AGE-RELATED COGNITIVE AND MOTOR DECLINE.[4]

For extra bulk and texture, add 3½ ounces/100g cooked and seasoned green lentils and a tangle of sautéed thinly sliced red onion (add 159 calories, or 80 per serving).

NO-POTATO SALADE NIÇOISE

CALORIE COUNT: 253

This is one of my favorite fallback recipes, stacked with lots of interesting morsels and a little French Riviera sophistication. If you are entertaining on a fast day—and I don't see any reason not to, as long as you can forgo the goblets of wine—this makes a gorgeous glamour plate for a party. Simply multiply the quantities according to how many friends show up, and perhaps serve with grilled tuna rather than the canned variety.

Serves 2

One 7-ounce/200g fresh tuna steak or one 6-ounce/170g can solid white tuna in water, drained
Tender salad leaves (such as green and red leaf, oak leaf, baby red romaine, baby arugula)
7 ounces/200g thin green beans, steamed or boiled and refreshed
1 hard-boiled medium egg, cooled, peeled, quartered
Scant 2 ounces/50g cherry tomatoes, halved
8 black olives
A squeeze of lemon juice
1½ teaspoons good-quality olive oil
Salt and pepper
2 anchovy fillets (optional)
Lemon wedges, for serving

If using fresh tuna, season and grill in a hot cast-iron pan till cooked to your liking. Allow to rest. Assemble the leaves, green beans, egg, tomatoes, and olives decoratively in a bowl. Dress with lemon juice and olive oil. Place the tuna on top, season, and garnish with anchovy fillets (if using) and lemon wedges.

NB

ONE PORTION DELIVERS OVER 1 OUNCE OF PROTEIN AND A HOST OF HEALTH-BOOSTING PHYTOCHEMICALS.

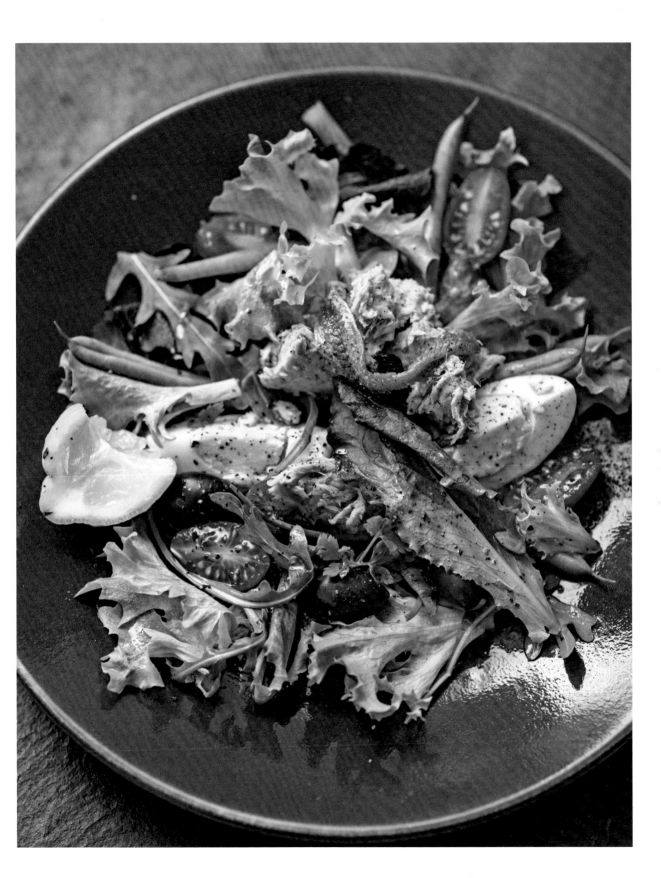

WATERCRESS, ORANGE, AND ALMOND SALAD WITH POPPY SEED DRESSING

CALORIE COUNT: 287

You could eat an entire two pounds of watercress for a mere 110 calories—better still, a study recently found that eating 3 ounces daily increases levels of the cancer-fighting antioxidants lutein and beta-carotene.[5] Okay, so that's a lot of watercress, but it does mean it's worth eating as often as possible. I'm more entranced by its wild taste: dense, delicious, and—it seems to me—the precise flavor I imagine when I think of green.

Salad

A generous handful of watercress, tough stems removed
1 orange, peeled and segmented
10 blanched almonds, coarsely chopped

Dressing

1 teaspoon Dijon mustard
2 teaspoons red wine vinegar
½ teaspoon honey
2 teaspoons canola oil
2 teaspoons poppy seeds
Salt and pepper

Combine the salad ingredients. Drizzle with the dressing and serve.

NB

YOU'LL GET TWICE THE RDA FOR VITAMIN C FROM THIS SALAD—NOT A BAD THING; IF YOUR BODY NEEDS EXTRA YOU'LL RETAIN IT; IF NOT, IT'S EXCRETED.

You may wish to add

- A handful of sliced cremini mushrooms (add 5 calories)

- Slivers of fennel, a sprinkle of fennel seeds, and sprigs of mint (add 3 calories)

- Or swap the watercress for raw spinach or finely chopped kale and add thin slices of red onion and 1 teaspoon pine nuts (add 34 calories)

PINK LEAVES, RED FRUITS, AND BLUE CHEESE

CALORIE COUNT: 333

It's probably worth eating this salad for the title alone—but it also brings some fine fast day ingredients to your plate. Look for russet-skinned pears, and keep the skin on (a great source of fiber). Pears, like apples, have a relatively low GL—they score a respectable 4, about the same as a fresh fig. The suggestion of Stilton cheese here completes the equation for this well-loved dish: pear + walnuts + blue cheese = delicious.

Serves 2

1 head endive (red Treviso or Castelfranco makes it pretty)
A handful of radicchio leaves
1 red Bartlett pear, quartered, cored, sliced, and tossed with a squeeze of lemon to prevent discoloration
1 fresh purple or brown turkey fig, cut into eighths
Scant 2 ounces/50g walnut halves
1 tablespoon good-quality balsamic vinegar
1 tablespoon good-quality olive oil
Salt and pepper
Pomegranate seeds, for serving
Scant 2 ounces/50g good-quality blue cheese, such as Stilton, Maytag, or Rogue Creamery blue

Assemble the endive and radicchio leaves in a bowl, then scatter in the pear, fig, and walnuts. Dress with the vinegar and olive oil. Season, then scatter with pomegranate seeds and a snowy crumble of cheese.

NB

PEARS ARE EASY TO DIGEST AND ONE OF THE LEAST ALLERGENIC FOODS AROUND.

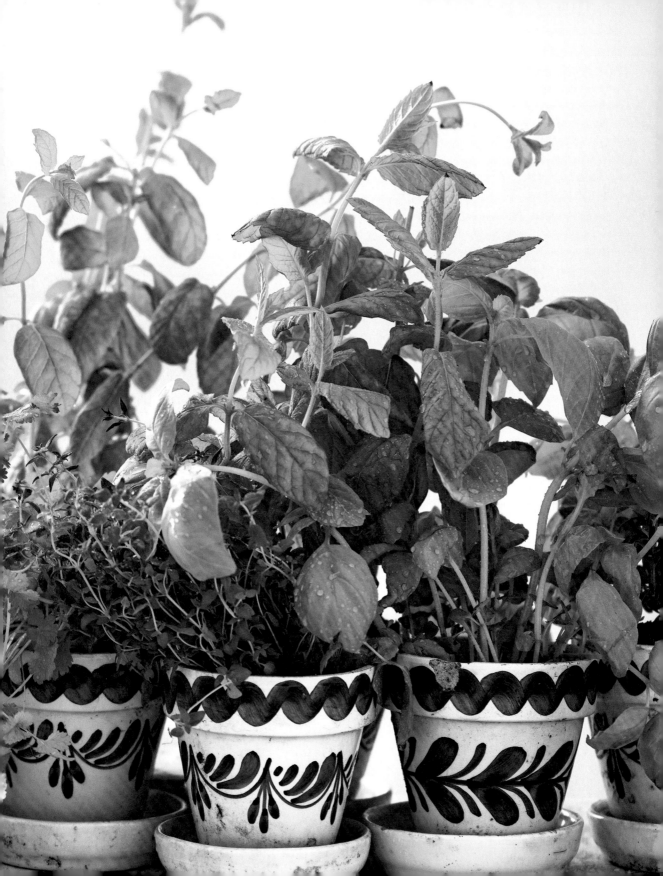

CHAPTER TWELVE

flavor savior condiments

Fast day food always needs a jolt of flavor, so here are ways to add a potent boost of taste to your plate. Each recipe makes plenty, and calorie counts are for 1 tablespoon. In many of these recipes, the rest will keep happily in the fridge for a day or two.

CILANTRO AND CHILE SAUCE

CALORIE COUNT PER TABLESPOON: 19

3 cloves garlic, chopped
1 teaspoon light brown sugar
1 teaspoon minced fresh ginger or galangal
1½ teaspoons tamarind paste
2 teaspoons lime juice
A large handful of fresh cilantro leaves, chopped
1 or 2 fresh chiles, chopped (seed if you prefer less heat)
2 tablespoons water

Blend in a mini food processor, or with a stick blender, and serve a spoonful alongside grilled white fish. Store in the fridge in a closed container for no more than a few days.

GREEN HERB RELISH

CALORIE COUNT PER TABLESPOON: 38

Scant 2 ounces/50g mixed fresh herb leaves (flat-leaf parsley, basil, mint, and chives)
1½ tablespoons capers, rinsed
2 cloves garlic, finely chopped
Juice of 1 lemon
2 tablespoons extra virgin olive oil

Blend in a mini food processor and serve.

SALSA FIVE WAYS

A fine way to bring a jolt of low-calorie flavor to a fast day plate. A good salsa is all about the balance and freshness of ingredients, and it needn't rely on the classic union of tomatoes and onion. Salsa simply means sauce, so you can riff on the theme.

Classic Tomato

CALORIE COUNT PER TABLESPOON: 4

10 ounces/300g ripe tomatoes, peeled, seeded, and chopped
½ red onion, finely chopped
1 tablespoon white wine vinegar
2 teaspoons lime juice
A pinch of sugar
A pinch of red pepper flakes
A few fresh basil leaves, torn
Salt and pepper

Mix everything in a small bowl. Use immediately, as this does not keep well.

Roasted Tomato with Green Chile

CALORIE COUNT PER TABLESPOON: 10

3 ripe tomatoes, halved and seeded
1 or 2 whole green chiles
½ small onion
2 cloves garlic, finely chopped
¼ teaspoon sugar
Coarse sea salt and pepper
3 tablespoons chopped fresh cilantro
A squeeze of lemon juice

Preheat the oven to 400°F. Place the tomatoes (cut side down), chiles, and onion (cut side down) in a small baking pan. Roast till just charred. When cooled, halve the chiles and scoop out the seeds. Place the chiles in a mortar and pound with a pestle or grind in a mini food processor and add the garlic, sugar, and salt. Add the tomatoes and crush with a fork or pulse briefly till combined. Stir in the cilantro, lemon juice, and onion, and season with pepper.

Fennel and Cucumber

CALORIE COUNT PER TABLESPOON: 5

1 seedless cucumber, peeled, cored, and diced
1 bulb fennel, finely diced
½ red onion, finely diced
A handful of fresh cilantro, chopped
1 tablespoon white wine vinegar
1 tablespoon lemon juice
Salt and pepper

Mix everything in a small bowl. Use immediately, as this does not keep well.

Watermelon

CALORIE COUNT PER TABLESPOON: 6

7 ounces/200g watermelon, seeded and finely diced
2 scallions (green onions), finely chopped
1 yellow bell pepper, seeded and finely diced
A handful of fresh cilantro, chopped
Juice of ½ lime
Salt and pepper

Mix everything in a small bowl. Use immediately, as this does not keep well.

Watercress Salsa Verde

CALORIE COUNT PER TABLESPOON: 31

3 ounces/85g watercress, thick stems removed
2 tablespoons chopped fresh basil
1 clove garlic, chopped
2 tablespoons lemon juice
2 teaspoons olive oil

Blend in a mini food processor and serve alongside poached salmon fillets.

CUCUMBER RAITA

CALORIE COUNT PER TABLESPOON: 6

An Indian classic designed to calm, cool, and cleanse the palate. Do eliminate as much water as possible from the cucumber—you'll get a better raita that way.

1 large seedless cucumber
Salt and pepper
1 heaping cup/250g unflavored low-fat yogurt
Chopped fresh mint leaves

Peel the cucumber and shave into long ribbons using a vegetable peeler. Discard the central core. Place cucumber strips in a colander with a scattering of salt. Leave to stand for 30 minutes, then squeeze out excess water using paper towels. Mix the cucumber with the yogurt, stir in the mint, season, and serve alongside any fast day curry.

TZATZIKI

CALORIE COUNT PER TABLESPOON: 6

The Greek version of raita, familiar from meze plates. The addition of crushed garlic brings a Mediterranean hum to the proceedings. Perfect with barbecued vegetable kebabs.

½ cup/100g unflavored low-fat yogurt
2 teaspoons minced garlic
½ small seedless cucumber, peeled, cored, and diced
Chopped fresh cilantro
Chopped fresh mint leaves
A squeeze of lemon juice
Salt and pepper

Mix everything in a small bowl. Use immediately, as this does not keep well.

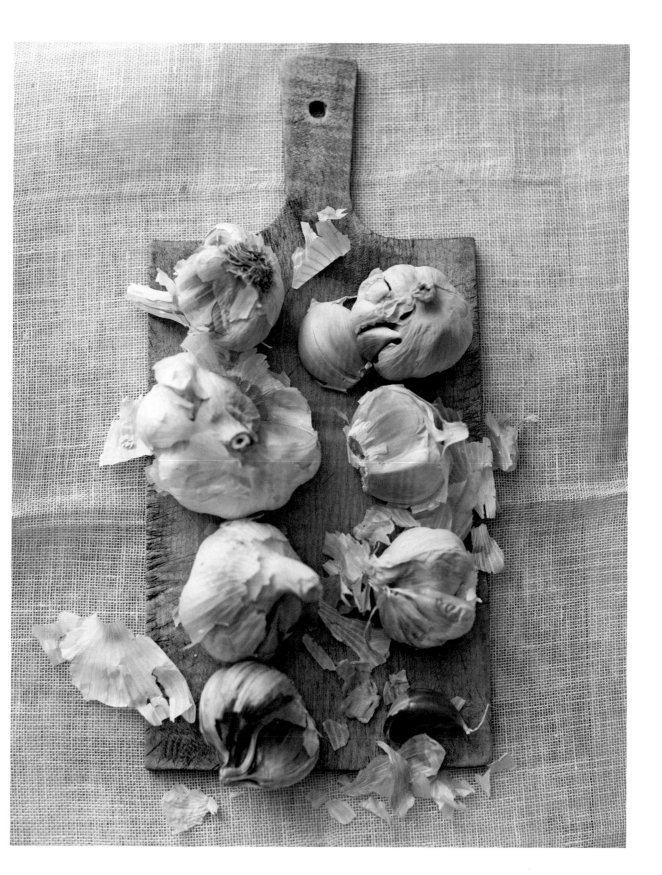

PESTO FOUR WAYS

We have come to love pesto, the classic Italian green sauce—nutty, cheesy, and garlicky. You can of course buy it fresh from the supermarket (avoid the jars, though—you'll be eating unnecessary preservatives). But making it at home is so easy. The roasted red pepper pesto will save you calories, as it dispenses with the cheese and nuts.

Green Classic

CALORIE COUNT PER TABLESPOON: 71

3 handfuls fresh basil leaves
½ clove garlic
1½ ounces/40g pine nuts
1 ounce/30g Parmesan cheese, grated
1 tablespoon good-quality olive oil
1 teaspoon lemon juice
Salt and pepper

Gently pulse the ingredients in a food processor, adding a little more oil if necessary to achieve the desired consistency. Drizzle over grilled zucchini and asparagus.

Red and Fiery

CALORIE COUNT PER TABLESPOON: 90

1 clove garlic, chopped
Scant 1 ounce/25g pine nuts
7 ounces/200g sun-dried tomatoes (drained well if oil-packed)
1 red chile, seeded and coarsely chopped
A handful of fresh flat-leaf parsley
Scant ½ cup/100ml good-quality olive oil
Scant 1 ounce/25g Parmesan, finely grated
Salt and pepper

Pulse the ingredients in a food processor, keeping the paste coarse and adding a little more oil if necessary to achieve the desired consistency.

Roasted Red Pepper

CALORIE COUNT PER TABLESPOON: 12

2 cloves garlic, peeled
4 red bell peppers, roasted till soft and charred, peeled, stemmed, and seeded
3½ ounces/100g fresh basil leaves
2 tablespoons good-quality olive oil
Salt and pepper

Blitz in a food processor till smooth.

Parsley and Pumpkin Seed

CALORIE COUNT PER TABLESPOON: 76

1 clove garlic
3½ ounces/100g flat-leaf parsley
1 teaspoon salt
3 tablespoons/50ml good-quality olive oil
Scant 2 ounces/50g shelled pumpkin seeds (pepitas)

Blitz to a coarse paste in a mini food processor.

THREE GOOD DRESSINGS

A salad without dressing is a marriage without love—you can get by, but no one's particularly happy. These three are well worth having in your repertoire, to be used sparingly.

Tomato Vinaigrette

CALORIE COUNT PER TABLESPOON: 13

14 ounces/400g ripe tomatoes, peeled and seeded
A pinch of sugar
2 tablespoons white wine vinegar
2 tablespoons good-quality olive oil
Salt and pepper

Puree in a blender. Serve with grilled fish or dark leafy salads.

Simple Lemon, Garlic, and Herb

CALORIE COUNT PER TABLESPOON: 112

2 tablespoons good-quality olive oil
1 to 2 tablespoons lemon juice
1 teaspoon Dijon mustard
1 clove garlic, crushed
Salt and pepper
Dried oregano or herbes de Provence, to taste

Whisk together. Serve with grilled chicken.

Asian Dressing

CALORIE COUNT PER TABLESPOON: 22

2 tablespoons soy sauce
2 teaspoons sesame oil
2 teaspoons minced fresh ginger
2 cloves garlic, crushed
2 teaspoons mirin
2 teaspoons lime juice
2 tablespoons cold water

Whisk together. Drizzle over crisp Asian salad vegetables.

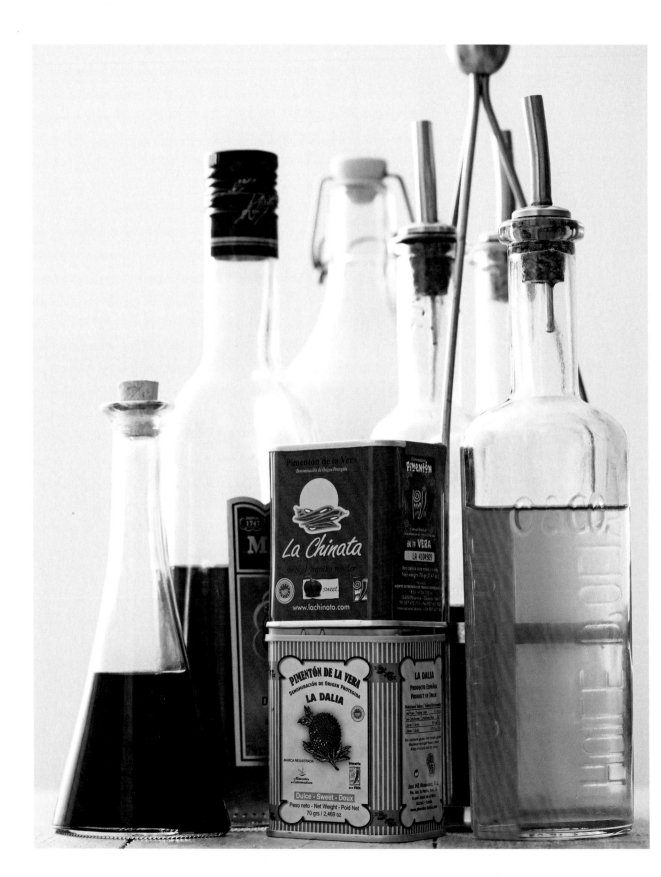

DRY RUBS

The key to brilliant fast day food is finding ways to impart deep, satisfying, interesting flavor without unnecessary calorie cost. While fats, oils, and sugars do tend to make everything taste very good indeed (it's why we're hooked), you can easily add depth and interest without resorting to butter and cream. These dry rubs are versatile and do the job admirably, rubbed into any lean meat or fish or sprinkled on vegetables—or how about grilled haloumi cheese? Make them fresh to get maximum glory, though of course they'll keep well in an airtight jar.

Italian Fennel and Thyme

1 tablespoon fennel seeds
1 tablespoon dried thyme
½ teaspoon celery seeds
1 clove garlic
Salt and pepper

Indian Masala

Toast the spices before grinding.

1½ teaspoons fennel seeds
1½ teaspoons coriander seeds
1½ teaspoons cumin seeds
1 teaspoon ground fenugreek
1 cardamom pod
1 small piece cinnamon bark
Salt and pepper
Cayenne pepper, to taste

Asian

1 tablespoon ground coriander
1 tablespoon red pepper flakes
1 tablespoon minced lemongrass
1 tablespoon ground ginger
1 tablespoon Kaffir lime leaves

Tunisian

Good with chicken and roasted vegetables.

1 tablespoon garlic powder
1 tablespoon ground cumin
1 tablespoon ground coriander
1 tablespoon ground ginger
1 tablespoon paprika
1 tablespoon ground turmeric
1 tablespoon ground cinnamon
1 tablespoon black peppercorns
Cayenne pepper to taste
Grated zest of ½ lemon

Ras al Hanout

Great on lean steak or chicken.

2 teaspoons ground ginger
2 teaspoons ground cardamom
2 teaspoons ground mace
1 teaspoon ground cinnamon
1 teaspoon ground allspice
1 teaspoon ground coriander
1 teaspoon ground nutmeg
1 teaspoon ground turmeric
½ teaspoon ground black pepper
½ teaspoon ground white pepper
½ teaspoon cayenne pepper
½ teaspoon ground anise seeds
¼ teaspoon ground cloves

Creole Blackening Rub

2 teaspoons pink peppercorns
2 teaspoons black peppercorns
2 teaspoons garlic powder
2 teaspoons smoked paprika
2 teaspoons cayenne pepper
2 teaspoons sea salt
2 teaspoons dried oregano
2 teaspoons dried thyme
½ teaspoon brown sugar
½ teaspoon ground cumin
A grating of nutmeg

Egyptian Dukkah

1 tablespoon roasted blanched hazelnuts
1 tablespoon toasted sesame seeds
1 teaspoon toasted coriander seeds
1 teaspoon toasted cumin seeds
1 teaspoon black peppercorns

Texas Dry Rub
Great on chicken.

1 clove garlic
2 teaspoons red peppercorns
2 teaspoons ground cumin
2 teaspoons mustard seeds
½ teaspoon salt
½ teaspoon pepper
½ teaspoon chili powder
½ teaspoon paprika

Grind all the ingredients together with a mortar and pestle or in a mini food processor.

WET RUBS

Think of these as massages. Most contain a little oil, but even so, they are a fine way to introduce fire and zing without too great a calorie cost.

Lemon Zinger

Marinate chicken, fish, or shellfish, grill or broil, and serve with plenty of lemon-dressed leaves.

Grated zest and juice of 1 lemon
2 tablespoons olive oil
1 clove garlic
Leaves from a handful of fresh thyme
A grating of nutmeg
Salt and pepper

Memphis BBQ

Smear on lean pork loin. Leave to marinate for an hour or more before barbecuing.

1 tablespoon smoked paprika
1½ teaspoons dry mustard
2 teaspoons cayenne pepper, or to taste
1 tablespoon maple syrup
Salt and pepper

Jerk

Rub well over a whole chicken. Roast or barbecue till cooked through.

2 teaspoons ground allspice
1 teaspoon ground cinnamon
A grating of nutmeg
1¼-inch piece fresh ginger, peeled and finely chopped
3 cloves garlic, crushed
2 shallots, finely chopped
1 tablespoon chile puree
1 tablespoon lime juice
1 tablespoon olive oil
Leaves from a handful of fresh thyme
Salt and pepper

North African Chermoula

This makes a great base for any tagine.

A handful of fresh cilantro, chopped
2 cloves garlic, peeled
1 tablespoon paprika
1½ teaspoons ground cumin
1 teaspoon coarse sea salt
½ teaspoon ground ginger
Cayenne pepper, to taste
A pinch of ground saffron
1 tablespoon peanut oil

Grind all ingredients together with a mortar and pestle or in a mini food processor.

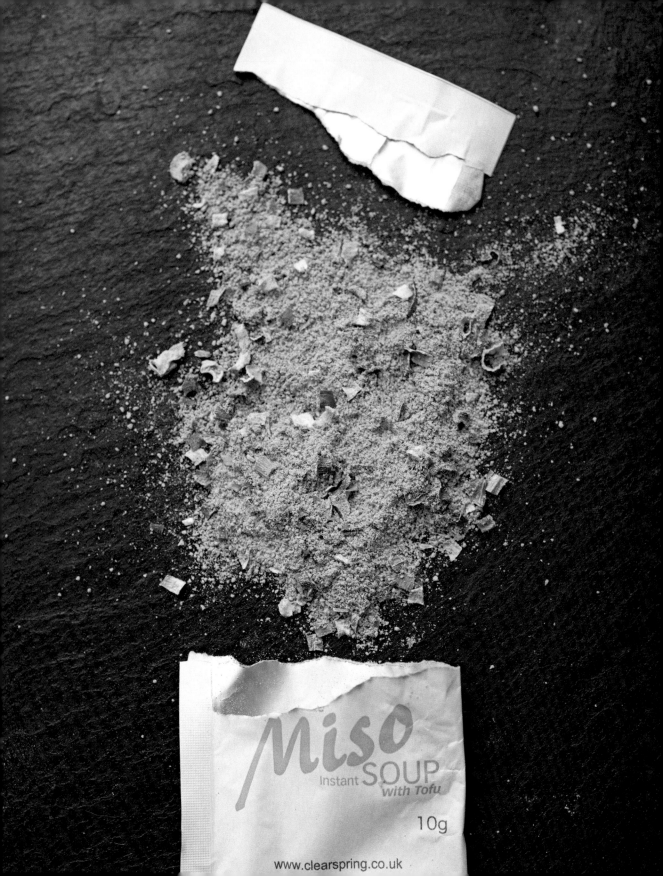

Miso
SOUP
Instant with Tofu

10g

www.clearspring.co.uk

fast day snacks

There's little point in grazing on a fast day—it would soon eliminate the point of the exercise. But some people need a little lift, particularly in the early days when your appetite is adjusting to the new regimen. If tummy rumbles get the better of you, reach for one of these Super Snacks. It's best to avoid easy carbs and go instead for fresh, raw ingredients. Have them prepped and handy in the fridge. Nuts, though high in calories, are full of protein and good fats, and just a few will help you feel full.

- A handful of almonds, 80 calories for 6

- Crudités: carrot, celery, and cucumber sticks; raw bell pepper strips; watercress; radishes; cherry tomatoes—about 40 calories per serving (a medium bowlful)

- 1 tablespoon hummus, 56

- 10 fresh strawberries, 30

- 2 ounces/60g pitted cherries, 23

- 3½ ounces/100g blackberries, 25

- 3½ ounces/100g blueberries, 57

- 1 tablespoon cottage cheese, 40

- 1 ounce/25g Edam or reduced-fat cheddar cheese, 85

- 1 cup/10g air-popped popcorn, 59

- 10 shelled pistachios, 60

- 1 apple, sliced, including skin and core, with a squeeze of lemon juice, 48

- 2¼ ounces/60g plain edamame, steamed and served warm with a little coarse sea salt, 84

- 1 medium hard-boiled egg, 75 calories

- 2 hard-boiled quail eggs, 60

- 1 tablespoon shelled pumpkin and/or sunflower seeds, 90

- A few frozen grapes, 60

- 1 sugar-free gelatin snack, 10

- 1 cup of miso soup, 32

- Something tasty or crunchy from the fridge. A bite of pickled guindilla pepper, cucumber, or jalapeño; or a few cornichons, 8 to 10 calories

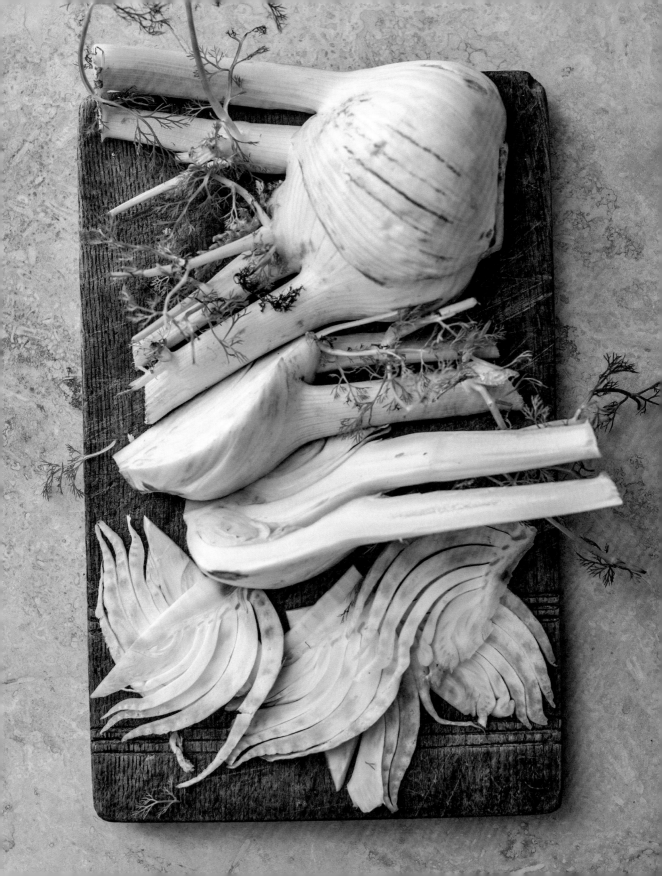

meal plans

500-CALORIE MEAL PLANS FOR 4 WEEKS

DAY #	BREAKFAST	MEAL CAL	SUPPER	MEAL CAL	TOTAL CAL FOR DAY
DAY 1	Poached Egg with Spinach, Mushroom, and Tomato (page 31)	124	Roasted Sardines (page 138)	399	523
DAY 2	High-Energy Breakfast (page 39)	246	Skinny Bouillabaisse (page 180)	163	409**
DAY 1	Yogurt with Plum (page 24)	264	Lo-Lo Meatballs (page 154)	264	528
DAY 2	Spiced Pear Porridge (page 43)	286	Masala Chicken, Spinach, and Raita (page 146)	219	505
DAY 1	Fluffed Shrimp Omelet (page 36)	207	Greek Salad (page 195)	229	436**
DAY 2	Strawberries with Ricotta (page 20)	120	Couscous with Lemon Tofu (page 70)	355	475*
DAY 1	Soft-boiled Egg with Asparagus Spears (page 19)	90	Tuna with Chile Green Beans (page 129–30)	367	457*
DAY 2	Muesli with Cherry Yogurt (page 38)	223	Chicken Puttanesca (page 152)	247	470*

*Allowance for 1 small piece of fruit (apple, tangerine, pear, 3½ ounces strawberries) or drop of milk in tea or coffee.

**Allowance for additional small snack (10 almonds).

600-CALORIE MEAL PLANS FOR 4 WEEKS

DAY #	BREAKFAST	MEAL CAL	SUPPER	MEAL CAL	TOTAL CAL FOR DAY
DAY 1	Yogurt with Plum (page 24)	264	Hot Thai Stir-fry (page 91)	341	605
DAY 2	Wilted Spinach Omelet (page 58)	297	Harissa-Spiked Chicken (page 148)	300	597
DAY 1	Shakshouka (page 32)	178	Grilled Chicken (page 160)	416	594
DAY 2	Spiced Pear Porridge (page 43)	286	Lightweight Cottage Pie (page 151)	243	529**
DAY 1	High-Energy Breakfast (page 39)	246	Lemon-Scented Chicken with Roasted Veggies (page 149)	287	533**
DAY 2	Lean Eggs (2) and Ham (page 20)	178	Charred Squid (page 137)	369	547*
DAY 1	Scrambled Eggs with Smoked Salmon (page 28)	303	Tuna Fagioli (page 132)	286	589
DAY 2	Muesli with Cherry Yogurt (page 38)	223	Warming Stew (page 159)	385	608

* Allowance for 1 small piece of fruit (apple, tangerine, pear, 3½ ounces strawberries) or drop of milk in tea or coffee.

** Allowance for additional small snack (10 almonds).

Fast Day Calorie Countdown

CALORIES	RECIPE	PAGE
4	Classic Tomato Salsa	206
5	Fennel and Cucumber Salsa	207
6	Cucumber Raita	208
6	Watermelon Salsa	207
10	Roasted Tomato Salsa with Green Chile	207
12	Roasted Red Pepper Pesto	210
13	Tomato Vinaigrette	211
19	Cilantro and Chile Sauce	205
22	Asian Dressing	211
31	Watercress Salsa Verde	207
38	Green Herb Relish	206
43	Summer Cucumber Salad with Dill	185
48	Fragrant Pho	163
52	Fennel, Cucumber, and Radish Salad with a Citrus Vinaigrette	186
53	Oysters with Mignonette	103
54	Clear Tofu Broth	164
58	Roasted Red Pepper Soup	165

CALORIES	RECIPE	PAGE
70	Bloody Mary Soup	168
71	Green Classic Pesto	210
72	Shaved Fennel and Orange Salad	68
76	Parsley and Pumpkin Seed Pesto	210
78	Miso Soup	41
87	Red Velvet Soup	163
88	Strawberries with Reduced-Fat Cottage Cheese, Black Pepper, and Balsamic	20–21
90	Red and Fiery Pesto	210
90	Soft-boiled Egg with Asparagus Spears	19
90	Steamed Salmon	42
91	Summertime Special Soup	166
93	Carrot and Ginger Soup	167
93	Tamagoyaki (Rolled Omelet)	41
100	Bloody Mary Soup with Vodka	168
102	North African Spring Vegetable Broth	170
102	Spinach, Sorrel, and Nutmeg Soup	171
107	Red Velvet Soup with Breadstick	166
108	Everything-from-the-Garden Soup	172
110	Asparagus Salad with Red Onion and Grilled Mushroom	187
112	Simple Lemon, Garlic, and Herb Dressing	211

CALORIES	RECIPE	PAGE
185	Watermelon, Fresh Fig, and Prosciutto	22
190	Red Tomato Dahl	81
191	Spicy Edamame	77
195	Ceviche with Cilantro Salad	106
195	Lime Chicken Salad, Szechuan Style	145
196	Sashimi with Wasabi and Pickled Ginger	54
196	Tapenade, Pine Nut, and Marjoram Tortilla Pizzetta	55
196	Whole Baked Sea Bass with Lemongrass	114
199	Chicken Masala Style with Raita	146
199	Standby Veggie Chili with a Taco Shell	48
203	Mozzarella and Pesto Tortilla Pizzetta	55
205	Bagna Cauda with Grilled Vegetables	84
206	Smoked Trout and Celery Root with Horseradish Cream	69
207	Fluffed Shrimp Omelet	36
207	Poached Egg (2) with Spinach, Portobello Mushroom, and Cherry Tomatoes	31
208	Steamed Mussels in a Light Tomato Broth	116
211	Smoked Fish with Spinach and Poached Egg	119
213	Baked Salmon with Peppered Kale	67
215	River Cottage Fish Parcels with Asian Spices	120
218	Feta and Black Olive Tortilla Pizzetta	55

CALORIES	RECIPE	PAGE
218	Red Lentil Tikka Masala	87
219	Chicken Masala Style with Raita and Spinach	146
219	Fresh Pea, Smoked Trout, and Dill Omelet	57
220	Baked Pork Tenderloin with Fennel	142
221	Green Papaya Salad with Chargrilled Beef	143
223	Fast Day Muesli with Fresh Cherry or Strawberry Yogurt	38
223	Sliced Apple with Cinnamon Dip	22
223	Simple Herb Salad with Warm Buttered Almonds	196
224	Green Lentil and Mint Dahl	82
225	Gravlax with Eggs	59
225	Leek and Lemon Shrimp	121
226	Skewered Monkfish with Balsamic Coleslaw	122
226	Crab and Artichokes	60
227	Chicken Teriyaki with Sesame Seeds	146
228	Fast Day Minestrone	182
229	Baked Salmon with a Tangle of Steamed Samphire	67
229	Greek Salad with Oregano and Mint	195
229	Hot Thai Stir-fry	91
230	No-Potato Salad Niçoise	200
230	Stir-fry Lemongrass Shrimp with Shirataki Noodles	124

CALORIES	RECIPE	PAGE
264	Lo-Lo Meatballs with Cavolo Nero	154
264	Yogurt with Plums, Blanched Almonds, and Agave Nectar	24
267	Chicken with French Tarragon and Lemon	147
268	White Fish Stew with Orange and Fennel	127
270	Spinach, Pea, and Lime Dahl	83
277	Green Gazpacho	175
279	Beauty Breakfast Shake	42–43
284	Zucchini, Goat Cheese, and Red Onion Omelet	57
284	Oatmeal with Jewel Fruits	27
286	Spiced Pear Porridge	43
286	Tuna Fagioli	132
287	Lemon-Scented Sticky Chicken with Roasted Veggies	149
202	Watercress, Orange, and Almond Salad with Poppy Seed Dressing	202
290	Chicken with Romano Peppers and Spinach	148
291	The Ginger Man's Grilled Chicken	160
297	Wilted Spinach, Fava Beans, and Pecorino Omelet	58
298	Spiced Baby Eggplant with Pomegranate Yogurt	96
298	Super Simple Eggplant Curry	62
298	Winter Waldorf Salad with Blue Cheese	197
299	Spiced Pear Porridge with Agave	43

CALORIES	RECIPE	PAGE
300	Swiss, Tomato, and Arugula Omelet	58
300	Harissa-Spiked Chicken	148
301	Red Pepper Hummus, Crudités, and Flatbread Dippers with Tahini	63
303	Red Vegetable Goulash	99
303	Scrambled Eggs with Smoked Salmon	28
309	Roasted Vegetables with Spiced Balsamic Glaze and Goat Cheese	94
312	Eastern Feta Salad	19
317	Seared Sesame Tuna	131
318	O'Kelly Fish	110
321	Poached Salmon with Green Bean Salad and Tomato-Anchovy Dressing	111
325	Red Vegetable Goulash with Kohlrabi and Radish Salad	99
327	Pesto Pronto Salmon with Ribbon Veggies	65
329	Lettuce Bowls with Shiitake Mushrooms and Hoisin Shredded Chicken	156
333	Cumin-Scented Turkey Burgers with Tomato Salsa and Corn on the Cob	141
333	Pink Leaves, Red Fruits, and Blue Cheese Salad	203
336	Seared Sesame Tuna with Soy-Mirin Dressing	129
345	Hot, Sweet, and Sour Tofu	101
345	Seared Sesame Tuna with Lemongrass Dipping Sauce	130
350	Herring with a Spiced Almond Crust	134
355	Couscous with Lemon and Mirin Tofu	70

CALORIES	RECIPE	PAGE
355	Super Simple Eggplant Curry with Rice	62
364	Allegra McEvedy's Bake-in-the-Bag Fish with Preserved Lemon Couscous	131
367	Seared Sesame Tuna with Chile Green Beans	130
369	Charred Squid with Lima Beans and Chile	137
375	Baked Salmon with a Warm Puy Lentil Salad	68
385	Warming Winter Stew	159
386	Red Lentil Tikka Masala with Rye Barley Roti	87
399	Roasted Sardines with Moroccan Spices	138
410	Shorbat Rumman	93
412	Spiced Baby Eggplant with Pomegranate Yogurt and Walnut Rice	96
438	Seared Sesame Tuna with Salsa Verde	130
457	Seared Mackerel on a Rainbow Salad	139

Resources

If your supermarket or local gourmet market doesn't stock some of the ingredients called for here, you can order them from these companies or get information over the Internet about where you can find them. Asian and South Asian markets, as well as Whole Foods, also carry many of the more "exotic" ingredients.

Amazon.com, for an astonishing range of goods.
Bob's Red Mill, bobsredmill.com, for grains and grain products. Check the Store Finder for a retail outlet near you.
D'Artagnan, dartagnan.com, for specialty meats and game.
Kalustyan's, kalustyans.com, for spices, legumes, grains, and tahini, harissa, tamarind, and curry pastes.
Penzeys Spices, penzeys.com, for unusual flavorings, spices, and spice blends.
The Spice House, thespicehouse.com, for spices and flavorings.
La Tienda, tienda.com, for Spanish ingredients including guindilla peppers and an array of paprikas.
The Spanish Table, spanishtable.com, for paprikas and peppers.
Your local farmers' markets and CSAs are the absolute best places for fresh, local, in-season produce. Check
localharvest.org/csa/ to find a community supported agriculture (CSA) subscription near you.

OVEN TEMPERATURES

FAHRENHEIT	CELSIUS	DESCRIPTION	FAHRENHEIT	CELSIUS	DESCRIPTION
225°F	110°C	Warm	350°F	180°C	Moderate
250°F	120°C	Warm	375°F	190°C	Moderately hot
275°F	140°C	Very low	400°F	200°C	Hot
300°F	150°C	Very low	425°F	220°C	Hot
325°F	160°C	Low	450°F	230°C	Very hot
325°F	170°C	Moderate			

Glossary

5:2 The intermittent fasting method devised by Dr. Michael Mosley: on two days, calories are cut to a quarter of the usual intake. On the five remaining days, you eat normally.

Alternate-day fasting (ADF) A version of intermittent fasting (IF), as developed by scientists including Dr. Krista Varady of the University of Illinois at Chicago.

Calorie cost The calories in any given food.

Calorie quota or **budget** The number of calories allowed on a fast day: 500 for women, 600 for men.

The FastDiet Michael and Mimi's 5:2 intermittent fasting method.

Fasting window The number of hours between meals on a fast day. Aim for a 12-hour window.

Glycemic index (GI) A measure of the effect of a carbohydrate on blood sugar relative to pure glucose (which scores 100).

Glycemic load (GL) A more useful measure, which takes into account how much of the carbohydrate is in the food:

$$GL = A \text{ score of under 10 is ideal on a fast day}$$

Intermittent fasting (IF) Occasional periods without food, or cutting back on calories for part of the time.

Recommended Daily Amount or **Recommended Dietary Allowance (RDA)** Also called Guideline Daily Amount or Recommended Daily Intake. The government-defined daily intake level of a nutrient considered to be sufficient for good health.

Acknowledgments

My thanks to the brilliant, brilliant Rebecca Nicolson and Aurea Carpenter at Short Books, and to Emmie Francis, Roz Hutchinson, Paul Bougourd, Catherine Gibb, Mary J. Jay, Katherine Stroud, and Sallie Coolidge—the publishing dream team.

To our U.S. publishers: Judith Curr, Sarah Durand, Benjamin Lee, Lisa Sciambra, Jeanne Lee, Kimberly Goldstein, Sybil Pincus, Daniella Wexler, and everyone else at Atria Books—thank you!

This book looks so delicious largely thanks to Romas Foord's heroic photographic sessions, along with stylist Polly Webb-Wilson and designer Georgia Vaux.

Thank you to Dr. Sarah Schenker for explaining the difference between thiamine and niacin, and for counting every last calorie in the book.

My thanks to the cooks, chefs, and food experts who have kindly donated recipes and good counsel to a cookbook rookie: Allegra McEvedy, Hugh Fearnley-Whittingstall, Ben McKellar, Sarah Raven, and Alex Renton.

And to my friends and family, always ready with a recipe and an interesting snippet about nettles or beetroot or exactly how to poach an egg: Debbie Spencer-Jones, Julie Spencer, Claire Denholm, Marcus Fergusson, and Penny Nagle.

Finally, thanks, as ever, to Nicola Jeal. And to Dr. Michael Mosley, without whom all of this would be academic.

Notes

CHAPTER ONE

1. K. Van Proeyen, K. Szlufcik, H. Nielens, K. Pelgrim, et al. "Training in the fasted state improves glucose tolerance during fat-rich diet." *Journal of Physiology*, November 2010.

   M.P. Harber, A.R. Konopka, B. Jemiolo, S.W. Trappe, et al. "Muscle protein synthesis and gene expression during recovery from aerobic exercise in the fasted and fed states." *American Journal of Physiology*, November 2010.

2. K.A. Varady, S. Bhutani, E.C. Church, and M. Kempel. "Short-term modified alternate-day fasting: a novel dietary strategy for weight loss and cardio-protection in obese adults." *American Journal of Clinical Nutrition*, November 2009.

   M.C. Klempel, S. Bhutani, M. Fitzgibbon, S. Freels, and K.A. Varady. "Dietary and physical activity adaptations to alternate day modified fasting: implications for optimal weight loss." *Nutrition Journal*, September 2010.

3. M.N. Harvie et al. "The effects of intermittent or continuous energy restriction on weight loss and metabolic disease risk markers: a randomised trial in young overweight women." *International Journal of Obesity*, May 2011.

CHAPTER TWO

1. Y. Yamamoto and R.B. Gaynor. "Therapeutic potential of inhibition of the NF-κB pathway in the treatment of inflammation and cancer." *Journal of Clinical Investigation*, January 15, 2001.

   M. Czaplińska, J. Czepas, and K. Gwoździński. "Structure, antioxidative and anticancer properties of flavonoids." *Postepy Biochemii* 58(3), 2012, 235–44.

   T.P.T. Cushnie and A.J. Lamb. "Recent advances in understanding the antibacterial properties of flavonoids." *International Journal of Antimicrobial Agents* 38 (2), 99–107.

2. J. Karppi et al. "Serum lycopene decreases the risk of stroke in men." *Neurology*, October 9, 2012, 1540–47.

3. V. Dewanto, X. Wu, K.K. Adom, and R.H. Liu. "Thermal processing enhances the nutritional value of tomatoes by increasing total antioxidant activity." *Journal of Agricultural and Food Chemistry,* April 2002.

4. E.E. Devore, J.H. Kang, M.M.B. Breteler, and F. Grodstein. "Dietary intakes of berries and flavonoids in relation to cognitive decline." *Annals of Neurology*, July 2012, 135–143.

5. R. Mattes. "Soup and satiety." *Physiology and Behavior.* January 2005, 739–47. See also M.E. Clegg, V. Ranawana, A. Shafat, and C.J. Henry. "Soups increase satiety through delayed gastric emptying yet increased glycaemic response." *European Journal of Clinical Nutrition*, January 2013, 8–11.

CHAPTER THREE

1. P. Schieberle. "Identifying substances that regulate satiety in oils and fats and improving low-fat foodstuffs by adding lipid compounds with a high satiety effect, "Perception of fat content and regulating satiety: an approach to developing low-fat foodstuffs," 2009–2012.

CHAPTER FOUR

1. A.C. Pappas, F. Karadas, P.F. Surai, et al. "Interspecies variation in yolk selenium among eggs of free-living birds: the effect of phylogeny." *Journal of Trace Elements in Medicine and Biology*, September 2006, 155–60.

2. F. Giampieri, S. Tulipani, J.M. Alvarez-Suarez, et al. "The strawberry: composition, nutritional quality, and impact on human health." *Nutrition*, January 2012, 9–19.

3. D. Schrenk. "Pectin, fat absorption and anti-carcinogenic effects." *Nutrition*, April 2008.

   J. M. Lattimer and M.D. Haub. "Effects of dietary fiber and its components on metabolic health." *Nutrients,* December 2010, 1266–89.

CHAPTER FIVE

1. N. Dhurandhar. "Egg protein for breakfast keeps you feeling full for longer."

2. RuiHai Liu. "Thermal processing enhances the nutritional value of tomatoes by increasing total antioxidant activity." *Journal of Agricultural and Food Chemistry*, April 2002.

3. M.E. Clegg, V. Ranawana, A. Shafat, and C.J. Henry. "Soups increase satiety through delayed gastric emptying yet increased glycaemic response." *European Journal of Clinical Nutrition*, January 2013.

4. M. Meydani. "Potential health benefits of avenanthramides of oats." *Nutrition Review*, December 2009.

CHAPTER SIX

1. B.B. Aggarwal and H. Ichikawa. "Molecular targets and anticancer potential of indole-3-carbinol and its derivatives." *Cell Cycle*, September 2005.
2. T.P. Domiciano et al. "Inhibitory effect of anethole in nonimmune acute inflammation." *Naunyn-Schmiedeberg's Archives of Pharmacology*, December 2012.

CHAPTER SEVEN

1. L. Cheskin. "Lack of energy compensation over four days when white button mushrooms are substituted for beef." *Appetite,* September 2008.
2. D.J. Jenkins et al. "Effect of legumes as part of a low glycemic index diet on glycemic control and cardiovascular risk factors in type 2 diabetes mellitus: a randomized controlled trial." *Archives of Internal Medicine,* October 2012, 1–8.

CHAPTER EIGHT

1. S.N. Stabler, A.M. Tejani, F. Huynh, and C. Fowkes. "Garlic for the prevention of cardiovascular morbidity and mortality in hypertensive patients." *Cochrane Database of Systematic Reviews* (online), August 2012.
2. C. Miglio, E. Chiavaro, A. Visconti, and V. Fogliano. "Effects of different cooking methods on nutritional and physicochemical characteristics of selected vegetables." *Journal of Agricultural and Food Chemistry*, December 2007.
3. A.T. Dinkova-Kostova and R.V. Kostov. "Glucosinolates and isothiocyanates in health and disease." *Trends in Molecular Medicine*, June 2012, 337–47.
4. B.Y. Kim et al. "Effects of *Asparagus officinalis* extracts on liver cell toxicity and ethanol metabolism." *Journal of Food Science*, September 2009.
5. D. Mozaffarian and E.B. Rimm. "Fish intake, contaminants, and human health: evaluating the risks and the benefits." *JAMA,* October 2006.

CHAPTER NINE

1. I.C. Ferreira, J.A. Vaz, M. H. Vasconcelos, and A. Martins. "Compounds from wild mushrooms with antitumor potential." *Anticancer Agents in Medicinal Chemistry,* June 2010, 424–36.

CHAPTER TEN

1. M.E. Clegg, V. Ranawana, A. Shafat, and C.J. Henry. "Soups increase satiety through delayed gastric emptying yet increased glycaemic response." *European Journal of Clinical Nutrition*, January 2013.
2. R.H. Mahmoud and W.A. Elnour. "Comparative evaluation of the efficacy of ginger and orlistat on obesity management, pancreatic lipase and liver peroxisomal catalase enzyme in male albino rats." *European Review for Medical and Pharmacological Sciences*, January 2013, 75–83.
3. M. Obulesu, M.R. Dowlathabad, and P.V. Bramhachari. "Carotenoids and Alzheimer's disease: an insight into therapeutic role of retinoids in animal models." *Neurochemistry International*, October 2011, 535–41.
4. M. Vafa, F. Mohammadi, et al. "Effects of cinnamon consumption on glycemic status, lipid profile and body composition in type 2 diabetic patients." *International Journal of Preventive Medicine*, August 2012, 531–36.
5. G. Gazzani, M. Daglia, and A. Papetti. "Food components with anticaries activity." *Current Opinion in Biotechnology*, April 2012, 153–59.
6. M.E. Clegg, M. Golsorkhi, and C.J. Henry. "Combined medium-chain triglyceride and chili feeding increases diet-induced thermogenesis in normal-weight humans." *European Journal of Nutrition*, November 2012.
7. L.J. Wylie, M. Mohr, et al. "Dietary nitrate supplementation improves team sport-specific intense intermittent exercise performance." *European Journal of Applied Physiology*, February 2013.

CHAPTER ELEVEN

1. M. Mansouri et al. "The effect of 12 weeks *Anethum graveolens* (dill) on metabolic markers in patients with metabolic syndrome: a randomized double blind controlled trial." *Daru* (Journal of Faculty of Pharmacy, Tehran University of Medical Sciences), October 2012.
2. G.B. Chainy, S.K. Manna, M.M. Chaturvedi, and B.B. Aggarwal. "Anethole blocks both early and late cellular responses transduced by tumor necrosis factor: effect on NF-κB, AP-1, JNK, MAPKK and apoptosis." *Oncogene*, June 2000, 2943–50.
3. L.F. Ferreira and B.J. Behnke. "A toast to health and performance! Beetroot juice lowers blood pressure and the O2 cost of exercise." *Journal of Applied Physiology*, March 2011.
4. E.E. Devore, J.H. Kang, M.M. Breteler, and F. Grodstein. "Dietary intakes of berries and flavonoids in relation to cognitive decline." *Annals of Neurology*, July 2012, 135–43.
5. C. Gill et al. "Watercress supplementation in diet reduces lymphocyte DNA damage and alters blood antioxidant status in healthy adults." *American Journal of Clinical Nutrition*, February 2012, 504–10.

Index

Page numbers in *italics* refer to illustrations.

About the Authors

MIMI SPENCER has written about body shape, diet, and food trends for more than twenty years—as a columnist for *Observer Food Monthly* magazine, and on *Waitrose Food Illustrated*, and as a feature writer for most national newspapers and magazines. But more than that, as she says, "I am a mother and a wife and a cook like you, wheeling my trolley around the supermarket, desperate for a bolt of inspiration about what to cook tonight. This book is as much a function of personal experience as professional know-how."

DR. SARAH SCHENKER is a registered dietitian and nutritionist who has served on both professional and government committees. She now combines her sports nutrition work, consulting for soccer teams including Tottenham Hotspur and Chelsea, with regular appearances on television and writing for scientific journals, as well as for newspapers, magazines, and websites. Sarah is married with two young sons—so she also has a busy mum's understanding of how best to feed a family. For *The FastDiet Cookbook*, Sarah used COMPEAT nutrition analysis software to complete the calorie calculations.

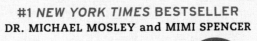
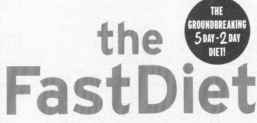